MUGGING

YOU CAN PROTECT YOURSELF

Liddon R. Griffith

A SPECTRUM BOOK

Prentice-Hall, Inc., Englewood Cliffs, New Jersey 07632

Library of Congress Cataloging in Publication Data

Griffith, Liddon R.
   Mugging.

   (A Spectrum book)
   1.   Self-defense.   2.   Crime prevention.
I. Title.
GV111.G68   613.6'6   78-4265
ISBN 0-13-604876-5
ISBN 0-13-604868-4 pbk.

To my Grandparents:

Mr. and Mrs. Kenneth Spencer

10   9   8   7   6   5   4   3   2   1

Printed in the United States of America

Photographs by Gregory Gore

PRENTICE-HALL INTERNATIONAL, INC., *London*
PRENTICE-HALL OF AUSTRALIA PTY. LIMITED, *Sydney*
PRENTICE-HALL OF CANADA, LTD., *Toronto*
PRENTICE-HALL OF INDIA PRIVATE LIMITED, *New Delhi*
PRENTICE-HALL OF JAPAN, INC., *Tokyo*
PRENTICE-HALL OF SOUTHEAST ASIA PTE. LTD., *Singapore*
WHITEHALL BOOKS LIMITED, *Wellington, New Zealand*

Acknowledgments

This book was developed from a course that I have taught for many years. During these years, I have benefitted from the influence of many people. For example, the many senior citizens who attended my classes shared their experiences with me. What I learned from these people has had a profound effect on the shaping of this book. Another important contribution has been made by the many youth gang members and former criminals who have helped me to understand mugging from the perpetrator's point of view. For this reason, I offer special thanks to Jose Rivera, Jesus and Natatalio Torres, Robert Sullivan, Francis Duggan, Peter Shivers, Robert Cruz, and Luis Ortiz. All of these people have helped me to attack the problems of violent crime against the person.

I also owe thanks to the members of the Housing Police Model Cities Police Cadet Program, headed by Lieut. David King and Sgt. James Brown. On many occasions, they have allowed me to use their cadets—particularly Nelson Falcon and Freddie Stokes—to assist the elderly. Thanks also to Gumersindo Martinez, Director of the South Bronx Model Cities.

A special thanks must be given to the many Senior Citizen Center Directors, especially Mrs. Catherine Jones, who stood by me when the program was in danger of being halted because of the employment cutbacks in New York City.

A hearty thanks must be offered to Commissioner Alice Brophy of the Department of the Aging in New York City, who has given me insight into the many problems facing the elderly and the handicapped. Thanks are also due to Ms. Clara Luna and Larry Minard, and other individuals in the Youth Employment Program. Also, I would like to express my gratitude to Court Employment, Loretta Brown and Carolyn Huggings, who have supported my efforts in finding jobs for the many youngsters I have worked with.

Special thanks are also due to Professor Richard Ward of John Jay College and Professor Joseph Peterson, formerly of John Jay College and now Director of the Forensic Science Foundation in Washington, D.C., both of whom encouraged the furthering of my program. I also thank the many members of the New York Housing Authority Police Department, especially those men assigned to the South Bronx Precinct. I thank

Capt. Joseph Irizarry for his contribution to this book and for having been my friend and supervisor for many years. His aide, Lieut. Charles Bentley, has also encouraged me in writing this book. From the inception of the program, I have been fortunate to have the support of Lieut. Arthur Brown, Lieut. James Ross, and Deputy Inspector Desmond Eaton.

The information in Chapter 6 was enriched by the assistance of Superintendent Robert R. Spillane, Principal James Gaddy, and Principal Lewis Lyman of the New Rochelle school system. They allowed me to visit their schools and gather pertinent information concerning youngsters and their many fears.

Chapter 4 contains an excerpt from the work of Dr. Martin Symonds and Chapter 9 includes an original case study by Dr. Estelle Fryburg. I am grateful to both persons for their contributions and I wish to thank Dr. Fryburg for voluntarily coming to the South Bronx to tutor the youngsters that I have been trying to help.

Judge Antonio Figueroa was kind enough to grant me the interview that appears in Chapter 10 and the New York Women Against Rape were considerate enough to review Chapter 5 and add an explanatory section. I am indebted to these people as I am to Jean Lax, Abbie Brownell, and Horace Orton for allowing me to reprint their letters of testimony.

I would also like to acknowledge the assistance of William Parmer of the Tenafly, N.J. Adult Education Program and of Linda Gottlieb, Eileen Eichenstein, and Alan Davis of Learning Corporation of America.

There are two people to whom I would like to express my particular gratitude: Mr. Gregory Gore and Mr. Ken Cashman. The first gentleman made it all happen. It was his interest in my work that was responsible for the publication of this book. But not only did he arrange to get my instructions into print, but he volunteered his services as a photographer. In so doing, he gave up several days of his own time to take the pictures that are such a crucial part of this book. I want to thank Greg for his fine work and for his friendship. I have come to value both.

There are really no words to express my gratitude to Ken Cashman. The complete manuscript in its current form is the work of Ken. He took my original ideas and some supplementary information and blended them into the book that you are going to read. In thanking Ken, I cannot over-look his wife, Evelyn. She fed us and looked after us through several long sessions. Shortly before the manuscript was completed, she gave birth to their third child.

Finally, and far from least, I give thanks to my wife, Dorothy, who has always stood by me, and to my four beautiful children: Liddon, Jr., Kevin, Wayman, and Ladonna.

Liddon R. Griffith

Contents

About the Author   *vii*

Foreword   *ix*

1. The Key to Safety   **1**

2. Knowing Your Assailant   **4**

The Model Mugger and the Predator, 4
The Desperate Mugger and the Professional, 5
Objectives of the Model Mugger, 6
Objectives of the Predator, 6
One Other Type of Mugger, 7

3. Avoiding Danger   **8**

When is Crime More Likely to Occur? 8
What We Do Wrong to Attract a Mugger, 12
What You Should Do If You Suspect Danger, 13
Crime Prevention in the Danger Zones, 15
Avoiding Danger at the Scene of a Crime, 29
What You Can Do to Help, 33

4. Fighting for Your Life   **38**

Knowing When to Use Force, 40
Three Rules to Remember, 42
Resisting the Unarmed Mugger, 44
Resisting the Mugger Who is Armed, 97
When You Think That You Can't Use Force, 128

5. Avoiding Rape   130

Profile of the Rapist, 132
Fighting Back Against the Rapist, 133
Getting Help After the Crime, 148

6. Self-Protection for Youngsters   152

Robberies in and Around the School, 152
Violence for Its Own Sake, 158
What Adults Can Do to Help, 160

7. What You Can Do at Home   162

Why Practice is Necessary, 163
The Amount of Practice Required, 164
The Methods of Practice, 165
Other Types of Preparation, 173
The Checklist, 174

8. Self-Evaluation   176

Test 1: Avoiding Danger, 176
Test 2: Fighting Off the Unarmed Mugger, 179
Test 3: Fighting Off the Mugger Who is Armed, 182
Test 4: Avoiding Rape, 185
Test 5: Self-Protection for Youngsters, 187

9. Conversations with Ex-Criminals   188

Peter Shivers, the Professional Mugger, 189
Jesus Torres, a Young Offender, 193
Francis Duggan, a Burglar, 196
Joey Rodriguez, a Delinquent, 200

10. A Final Thought   207

About the Author

I first met the author, who is known as "Griff" to his associates and friends, when we were appointed to the N.Y.C. Housing Authority Police Department in 1962. We were then police academy recruits. After we graduated, we did not see one another for five years. Then I returned to the academy as a recruit academic instructor, and Griff, who holds a black belt in jiu jitsu, was assigned to the academy as a recruit physical training instructor. From this second meeting, the two of us—and our families—became close friends.

In 1970, I was promoted to Lieutenant and reassigned as a C.O. of a federally funded Model Cities program for underprivileged youths that was being conducted by our department. Griff joined the staff as a physical training and academic instructor. In 1973, I was promoted to Captain and assigned to my present command. Griff was reassigned to the department's Community Relations Unit in Brooklyn. Following this assignment, he had two experiences that caused him to create his minicourse in self-protection.

First, his grandfather, who was then 82, was mugged twice in a relatively short period of time. After the second attack, while the signs of the recent beating were still evident, the older man visited his grandson. He chided Griff in the following manner: "You teach new police officers how to defend themselves—teach me to defend myself against my tormentors. I refuse to live in fear, a prisoner in my own apartment. There is no dignity in living like a hunted animal—help me to help myself. Teach me what you have so often taught your brother officers."

The second incident that prompted the creation of the minicourse happened while Griff was on the job. Sister Sally Butler—the director of a senior citizens community center in the Fort Greene area of Brooklyn—requested Griff's unit to present a crime prevention program. The unit C.O. agreed; a rudimentary program was

planned; and the entire unit was stunned when 500 senior citizens
· attended the seminar seeking assistance.

The seed was planted. Officer Griffith started to explore his
knowledge of self-defense to see if there were techniques that even
the aged or the handicapped could use against an attacker. He then
started to interview the tenants in the city housing projects and sur-
rounding areas. He found that many of these people were senior
citizens and many of them lived alone. Anxious to help these people,
he went to the courts, hospitals, and senior centers to talk with the
victims of crime. As he interviewed each victim, he asked himself
"What could this person have done to protect himself from his attackers?" Some of the answers to these questions were supplied by
muggers themselves. Griff spent several hours talking with former
criminals and, slowly, the concepts and techniques of a feasible self-
protection course were formalized.

Griff's next move was to approach his superiors in the department to suggest two things: (1) the creation of a course in self-
protection for all citizens and (2) the implementation of a "senior
citizens robbery unit." His suggestions were made two years before
the news media started to concentrate on attacks against the elderly.
While today public officials are striving to provide more protection
for senior citizens, at the time Griff's suggestions met with a cool
reception from his superiors in the department. Still, they grudg-
ingly 'gave him permission to teach the "self-protection course."
Within a few years, the demand for this course was so great that Griff
could not present his lecture to every group or organization that requested it. As a result, he started to write his instructions, so they
could be published in a book for everyone to read.

Now, the deed is done, and Griffith's self-protection course can
be shared by all. Hopefully, it will make you—the reader—more alert
and more secure in a society where crime is growing at a startling and
alarming rate.

My warmest wishes to the author, who is a firm friend and close
associate, in all his present and future endeavors.

Capt. Joseph Irizarry
C.O., South Bronx Precinct

Foreword

Although it is a sad commentary on our times that a book like *Mugging: You Can Protect Yourself* needs to be written at all, it is good to know that there are individuals like Liddon Griffith who have dedicated their lives to the prevention of one of society's most important concerns. Because it is an act usually directed at the elderly, or the weak, mugging is a crime that should concern all of us.

The crime of mugging has reached epidemic proportions; our urban centers have become breeding grounds for crime and our homes locked like fortresses, and our freedom curtailed by the ominous threat of a vicious attack. The reasons may be many, and the solutions far from satisfactory. As citizens we must address this threat as we would any disease by taking preventive action and by being prepared, should a mugger attack.

This book addresses the subject of mugging in a no-nonsense, realistic manner. The author is a 15-year veteran of the New York City Housing Police Department and has devoted the past five years to practical research on the problem of mugging—particularly, as it affects the elderly. His theories have been tested and have been proven to be effective, but we will never know how many people would have been victims had they not followed his advice.

Griffith's primary approach centers on the importance of preparation against attack. His basic premise, "self-protection," centers on the ability of an individual to overcome fear and take positive steps to deter an assailant. His approach is not foolproof (no human endeavor is), but it will reduce the probability of being mugged, and, more importantly, decrease the likelihood of serious injury. As the author notes, "The goal of self-protection is not to win a fight, but to escape from an opponent without getting hurt."

No doubt, many will approach this book with a good deal of skepticism. Having observed Officer Griffith on several occasions with a class of elderly "students," I know that his techniques can and do work. They are generally simple, but they are effective. They represent the results of research compiled over many years in interviews with both muggers and victims. This approach adheres to the basic principle that knowledge and practice are important in self-protection.

We live in a society which stresses education and knowledge. Few people would consider exposing themselves to a dangerous situation without some knowledge of the risks and an understanding of the steps necessary to avoid injury. We do not drive without understanding the rules of the road; we do not dive into the deep end of a pool without some instruction. Yet, few of us take the necessary time to try to avoid being the victim of a crime. When we are young and strong, the threat of crime is hardly considered, and as we grow older we do not consider the possibility of being a victim. Crime always seems to be directed at another person, at least until we are the victim.

The author offers a penetrating look at the various types of muggers; most of them are individuals who seek money or valuables and who do not use force unless necessary. Your reactions to a mugger can be the difference between a close call and serious injury.

In the following pages one finds not only good advice, but the answers (if there are answers) to the hundreds of questions that have been asked in Officer Griffith's classes. Unlike many so-called experts, he readily admits that he doesn't have the answers to all the questions. The answers he does offer are designed to minimize the risks. Many of the points he makes may not seem consistent with the views of others who profess to be crime prevention experts, yet Officer Griffith speaks from experience. His is not a textbook approach, but rather the results of having lived with the problem of mugging. His interest comes from a personal commitment which few authors may claim; a keen desire to help the victims in a meaningful and practical way.

One also finds in these pages some important points on how to help a neighbor who is in trouble and how cooperation can deter an assailant. Officer Griffith's common sense approach is most important in the inner-city where many people live virtually isolated lives while surrounded by thousands of people. We are all familiar with mugging cases in which neighbors simply observed another individual being attacked. We owe it to ourselves and to society to help our neighbors.

In these tumultuous times one cannot depend solely on the police for help. We must learn to help ourselves.

Officer Griffith has included several letters from individuals who were victimized after attending one of his classes. These are personal accounts by people who took time to learn about self-protection. The "case studies" used in the book represent the more common mugging situations. They offer the reader an opportunity to think about what action he or she might have taken during an attack.

Some readers may be troubled by the tactics suggested to ward off a hostile attack, but it must be remembered that a mugging is a life-or-death situation. When a decision is made to use force against a mugger, the victim must not hesitate. Practice in the use of force is crucial, for most of us are not raised to use dangerous force against another human being. The illustrations offered here are realistic as an aid to developing effective strategies in a mugging situation.

Having known and observed Officer Griffith for the past three years, I have come to heartily endorse his approach. He has taken a long time to write this book, and it comes from the heart. A great deal of thought and research have gone into it. I have watched Officer Griffith working with young and old men and women, all of whom learn with a genuine appreciation of his interest and commitment. Few are aware of his work with young people, many of them former muggers who changed their way of life because of Officer Griffith. A true student of human behavior, he is actively involved in helping to make our society a better place to live.

As Liddon said to me, "If it saves even one person from attack or serious injury, it will have been worth it."

Richard H. Ward
Vice President,
John Jay College of
Criminal Justice

1

The Key to Safety

The longest and most critical chapter of this text is entitled "Fighting for Your Life." This chapter tells you what to do if you are attacked. It reminds you over and over that your key to safety is knowing what you have available.

Right now there is a different key to your future well-being. That key is preparation—practicing the techniques of self-protection so you know how to react if you are the victim of a crime. This can be a form of life insurance. But, surprisingly, it is sometimes hard to convince people that preparation is worthwhile. They are skeptical for several reasons.

(1) One reason is fear. When you decide self-protection is necessary, you admit to yourself that your life may some day be in danger. Most people, however, do not want to face this possibility. They don't want to act out a mugging and pretend that they are the victim. Instead they would rather rationalize that there is a chance that they will never be mugged. It is possible that these people will be lucky, but there is no guarantee. No area is completely free from violence or crime. Even neighborhoods with low crime rates have their danger zones—places where a mugging is more likely to occur. If you were walking in a danger zone, would you rather be prepared or would you rather trust your luck? The choice seems obvious.

(2) Another argument against self-protection is that protection should be the job of the police and that too many muggers go free while too many innocent people are injured. It is easy to sympathize with this sentiment, but the people who raise this objection are thinking of what ought to be rather than what is. What's happening today is that crime is increasing and, unfortunately, so is the need for self-protection.

(3) Some people complain that practicing self-protection

1

makes them feel foolish. This is an honest reaction. But it is important to realize that a self-protection drill is like a fire drill or an air
raid drill. All three exercises are designed to save our lives in an
emergency. We learned to prepare for fire or air raids as children in
school. So we can participate in these drills without being embarrassed. The same should be true for the practice of self-protection.

(4) A busy schedule is another reason to pass up the study of
self-protection. It is true that many people work at two jobs and have
very little free time. But during the past year many busy people
found the time to learn a new dance step, a new card game, or maybe
some new tunes on a musical instrument. Learning self-protection
doesn't take long. If you can possiby find the time, it is a worthwhile
investment.

(5) Notice that I use the term "self-protection" instead of the
more common title "self-defense." When people hear the words "self-
defense," they usually expect a cram course in judo or karate. This
may discourage some people—especially the elderly—who feel that no
matter what they are taught, they will never be able to overpower an
attacker. To reach these people, it is important that I make a distinc-
tion. The goal of self-protection is not to win a fight, but to escape
from an opponent without getting hurt.

Sometimes this can only be accomplished by the use of force. For
this reason, I have demonstrated several techniques in Chapters 4
and 5. These techniques do not require great strength or agility.
They involve just a few simple moves. All of my techniques can be
used by elderly people as well as young people and by women as well
as men. To make this point emphatic, let me explain that my self-
protection course was first created for my grandfather. At the time,
he was half blind and 82 years old. Within a short while, he succeeded in mastering the entire course.

The use of force, however, is not all there is to self-protection.
For example, one of my students recently called me to say that she
was glad that she had had her purse snatched. I was puzzled by her
reaction. But she explained that giving up her money proved that
she had learned something in class. She had learned not to risk her
life to save money or material objects that were in her pocketbook.
Knowing when not to fight back is an important part of self-protection.

Another way of protecting yourself without using force is knowing how to react when you are in danger. A good example of this is a

woman who thought she was going to be mugged by a group of boys. She looked straight at the middle youth and said, "How is your mother? Tell her I said 'hello' when you get home." The boy was convinced that this woman really knew his mother and thus he left her alone.

The point is that you can protect yourself without being young or strong. Self-protection is a system that can be learned by almost anyone.

• • • From years of experience, I recognize that the idea of self-protection has to be sold—that people need to be convinced that preparation is really necessary. I hope that the arguments above have persuaded you. If so, you will be ready to agree that a few hours of reading and practice may well be your key to safety.

Assuming that you have recognized the need for preparation, you will still want to know if the techniques presented in this book really work. The answer is that they have worked in the past. (I have presented my lecture to over 5000 people and many of them have used my methods in a real-life situation. Ten people acknowledge that one of my techniques was responsible for saving their life.) What you will read in the following chapters is what I have learned from experience. There is no theory or guesswork involved.

My experience comes from my job as a policeman for the New York City Housing Authority and from my interviews with muggers and their victims. What I wanted to find out was what caused the muggers to commit their crimes, how did they choose their victims, and what incited the muggers to become violent. It was also important to learn how the actions of the victims affected the crime. I asked the victims to describe their behavior—were they passive, terror-stricken, did they try to resist?

The sum of this experience is now available to you in a few short chapters. I hope that you will never have to use what you are going to learn. But if you do, one of these lessons may be the key to your survival.

2

Knowing Your Assailant

When I present my lecture on self-protection, I am usually accompanied by a few associates. These people are not policemen or criminologists. They are muggers and former muggers.

The purpose of their being with me is to demonstrate the type of behavior that will attract the mugger. They also explain the actions that will cause the mugger to become violent. This information is helpful because what we are trying to do is avoid being hurt. If we can keep from being mugged, we have accomplished our goal. If we are mugged but not attacked, we are still fortunate.

Sometimes if we understand the mugger, we have a better chance of not being mugged or not being attacked. Why? Because we know how to behave when the mugger is around. Knowing how to act is as important as knowing how to use force. Remember in self-protection, the use of force is a last resort.

While it is important to understand muggers, it is impossible to group all of them in one class. No two individuals are alike. This applies to muggers as well as anyone else. For convenience, however, I will describe two general types of criminal: the model mugger and the predator.

THE MODEL MUGGER AND THE PREDATOR

Of the two types, the model mugger is by far the more common. In my opinion, over 90% of all muggers belong in this category. The goals of the model mugger are to get your money and to get away. Force is only used if it is necessary to accomplish one of these goals.

On the other hand, the predator wants more than money; he wants to hurt you. For this individual, the crime may be an excuse to become violent. If you find it is impossible to keep the predator from attacking, you will have to use the techniques that are shown in Chapter 4.

When I interview muggers, one of the questions I ask is "Why did you strike your victims?" The people I consider model muggers say they used force because they panicked or because their victims reacted too slow. The predators cannot give any reasons. To them, the violence is a part of the crime.

THE DESPERATE MUGGER AND THE PROFESSIONAL

Not all model muggers are alike. Within this class there are two smaller classes: the desperate mugger and the professional.

The desperate mugger commits his crime for a specific purpose. It may be to get money for drugs or possibly to get money to buy food for his family. The desperate mugger does not steal on a regular basis. He only resorts to crime when he has the need.

This type of criminal does not select his victim. He encounters the victim by chance. His usual method is to hide in a secluded place (maybe an alley or doorway) and to wait for the first person to come by. If you are alone and you are spotted by the desperate mugger, you are likely to be his prey.

The desperate mugger is a nervous individual—perhaps more nervous than the person being robbed. If you are approached by the desperate mugger, it is important to keep calm. Otherwise, this person may panic and become violent. Remember the desperate mugger is not a predator. He does not plan to use force. But he may strike. If he does, it is because of fear and not some inner anger.

The professionals are a different type of individual. They consider mugging their career. Many people in this category have become muggers because there is too much risk in other types of crime. For example, one person on my staff was a hijacker before he turned to mugging. He found there was less money to be made on the streets, but it was a lot safer. There was less chance of being caught by the authorities.

Unlike the desperate muggers, the professionals select their victims carefully. They look for signs that a person is carrying a large amount of money. They may even wait outside a bank or outside a large company on payday. The victim they choose is likely to be the person who is carrying the most.

The professional mugger does not plan to be violent. He uses force only if his safety is threatened or if force is necessary to complete the crime. In the next chapter, you will learn how to avoid this type of mugger. If, however, you do become his victim, the best thing to do is cooperate.

OBJECTIVES OF THE MODEL MUGGER

Before they commit a crime, criminals ask themselves two questions: "Can I commit this crime successfully?" and "Can I commit this crime without being caught?" The model mugger may word these questions differently. He may ask himself "Can I get the money?" and "Can I get away?" Getting the money and getting away are the objectives of the model mugger. He is not interested in hurting his victim. However, he may keep this a secret.

To get a person to cooperate, the model mugger may threaten to use force. He may flash a weapon or may hint that he has a weapon that he is going to use. Some muggers will pretend to be angry. They will shout and curse at the victim so that the victim is scared. This is just another device to get the victim to cooperate.

A large number of model muggers do not actually carry weapons. They know that if they are caught, the penalties will be more severe if they are armed. They also know that beating and robbing a victim is a more serious crime than just robbing him. Thus the smart mugger will avoid using force unless it is necessary to get away.

How does a victim know whether a mugger is bluffing or whether he intends to use force? Muggers do not wear labels saying "model" or "predator." Their objectives will not be clear until after the crime is completed. The answer to the question is that whether the mugger is bluffing or serious, you should always cooperate. Hand over what the mugger wants. If after you've done that the mugger is still threatening or still using force, you know it is time to react.

OBJECTIVES OF THE PREDATOR

The predator is also looking to commit a crime and get away. But this type of criminal has a third objective: to prove that he is superior to his victim. The predator may abuse, injure, or, in extreme cases, actually kill the person he is robbing. Of the two types of mugger, the predator is by far the more dangerous.

If you are approached by a predator, you must do your best to remain calm. Do not beg or plead with your assailant. This encourages the predator to become even more violent. If you have turned over your valuables and you are still in danger, it is probably time to react. The techniques in Chapter 4 are simple. They are often needed when you are dealing with this type of mugger.

ONE OTHER TYPE OF MUGGER

Recently, I have become aware of a type of a criminal who does not fit any of the patterns described above. I call this person the "status seeker." He is young and is probably a member of a gang or a part of a group of youngsters who admire crime. The status seeker may mug you for your money, but his real motive is to impress his friends.

Even among this group there are variations. The more active status seeker will commit a crime by himself or with one or two friends. Then, through his own bragging, he will let everyone know about his exploits. He is usually admired by younger teenagers and he may even teach them how to go out and mug. Among boys and girls his own age, this person is generally considered a hero.

Another type of status seeker does not take the initiative in committing a crime. He partakes in a robbery as part of a larger group. When the spoils are divided, his share may be very small.

This person does not commit a crime to impress his friends; he does it to win their approval. For his gang, mugging may not be very profitable, but it is a means of excitement.

What does this mean to you, the potential victim? Like other criminals, the status seeker is more likely to mug the lone individual, but he is not sensitive to clues that you are or are not carrying a large amount of money. He is more concerned with his own notoriety.

If you are approached by this individual and are slow to respond or do not cooperate, he will probably become violent. Failure to him means loss of image—in his own eyes and in the eyes of the neighborhood. To protect his image, this mugger will not hesitate to use force.

The important thing for you to remember is that although the status seeker is young, he is still dangerous. He should be treated with the same respect and caution that you would exercise in dealing with an adult criminal.

3

Avoiding Danger

Self-protection has two basic objectives: (1) to help you avoid being mugged and (2) to help you avoid being hurt if you *are* mugged.

The first goal is often referred to as *preventive* self-protection. It is a matter of recognizing dangerous situations and remembering to take simple precautions. The second goal—not getting hurt—can sometimes be accomplished without the use of force. This can often be done just by staying calm and remembering not to panic the mugger.

This chapter deals with prevention and with knowing how to act if you become the victim of a mugging. The use of force will not be discussed until Chapter 4.

WHEN IS CRIME MORE LIKELY TO OCCUR?

I can't promise that you ever will or will not be the victim of a mugging. But I do know that your chances of being mugged increase any time that you travel by yourself. Muggers prefer the lone target. They feel that there is less chance of meeting resistance and less chance of being identified—especially if the victim has been grabbed from behind.

This tells us two things. (1) When you are going out, there is safety in numbers. For this reason, many people make their shopping trips with one or more companions. (2) If you prefer to go out by yourself, you should recognize that this is a time for greater aware-ness. I suggest that you plan the route of your trip in advance. Try to travel along well-trafficked streets. Know what you have available along the way—for example, are there payphones, open stores, fire alarms, police stations, on-duty patrolmen? Try to think ahead of time about where you can get help if help should be necessary.

In areas where crime is prevalent, I recommend that people let a friend know when they are going out, where they are going, and when they expect to return. If the friend does not hear from them within a half hour of the time they were due back, the friend can phone places where they have been and, if necessary, can notify the police. This is a part of what I call the *buddy system*.

There are times of day, times of the week, and times of the year when outdoor crime is more likely to occur. I do not suggest that you keep yourself locked in your home during these times, but I do advise that you exercise greater precautions.

The more dangerous hours of the day are (1) night time, when the streets are dark and the mugger is less likely to be observed; (2) school hours, when the streets are empty because most young people are in class and most adults are at their jobs; and (3) from 5 to 7 P.M., when people are coming home from work and many of them are bringing home their pay. The third time is very lucrative for muggers on Thursdays and Fridays. Most people—civil service employees especially—are paid at the end of the week. Professional muggers know this and are most active on these days. Another time that is busy for the knowledgeable mugger is the beginning of the month. This is the time when senior citizens are receiving their social security checks. So many of these checks have been stolen that the government now offers to mail them directly to the bank.

Outdoor crime is heaviest during two seasons of the year: the summer, when more people are on the streets; and the holiday season, when people are out shopping and are carrying extra money. These are times to keep up your guard. It would be good if you could finish your shopping a month ahead of Christmas. There are less robberies then and the stores have a wider selection of merchandise. Many people try to buy their Christmas gifts ahead of time, but not too many succeed. If you are shopping in December, the important thing is to be aware.

I have mentioned that people who are out by themselves are prime targets of a mugger. People who carry pocketbooks are also likely targets. An experienced purse snatcher can grab a pocketbook and escape in a matter of seconds.

For this reason, it is a good idea to keep your purse in your apparel and to leave your pocketbook at home. If this is not possible, you should be careful to carry your pocketbook in the proper way. Do not let it dangle. A dangling pocketbook kept far from the body is a signal to any purse snatcher. It tells him that he can make an easy grab and an easy getaway. The way to carry your pocketbook is close to the body with the flap facing toward you (as shown in the photograph). Some authorities suggest that you carry your pocketbook in your hand or under your arm rather than by the straps. This may be effective, but most of today's pocketbooks are too big to be comfortably carried in this way.

Men should be careful not to carry a bulging wallet and not to keep their wallet in an outside pocket. The preferable places for a wallet are in the back pocket, which can be buttoned, or in the inside pocket of a jacket.

If you suspect pickpockets, there is a way of holding your wallet without attracting attention. Slip it into your front pocket and keep your hand in your pocket. This will not seem unusual since many men keep their hands in their front pockets.

This is similar to a technique that is used by policemen. When they suspect danger, they want to keep a hand on their gun, but they don't want to be conspicuous. Thus they hold the weapon in their front pocket instead of walking around with their hand on their holster.

This leads me to a short digression. In my classes, I am often asked, "How much money should a person carry?" and "Where can valuable possessions be hidden so they won't be taken?" There is no good answer to either question. People who raise the first question are afraid that if the mugger isn't satisfied with what they have he will become violent. But how much money is enough? It depends on the mugger's needs. If he needs five dollars, four will not be sufficient. If he needs 15 to 20 dollars for a fix, 10 will not be good enough. If he is the predatory type of mugger, it is possible that no amount will keep him from being violent.

What should you do if the mugger is not satisfied with what he has stolen? You will have to decide if the mugger is likely to hurt you and if force may be necessary. A good precaution may be to calmly apologize. Tell the mugger "I'm sorry that I don't have more. If I did, I would certainly give it to you." This may convince the mugger that you are sincere. It may calm him down so that he doesn't use force. When you take this approach, you are not begging. You are using a subtle technique to control the situation.

The other question is "Where can money be hidden?" This is also difficult to answer. I have heard of muggers who have found money in their victim's shoes. There are few places where you can

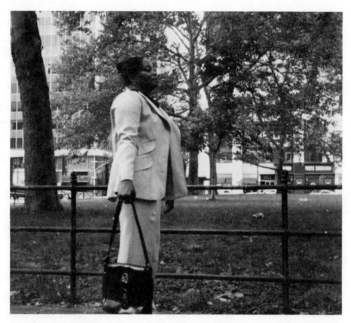

The wrong way to carry a pocketbook. The dangling bag is an invitation to the purse snatcher.

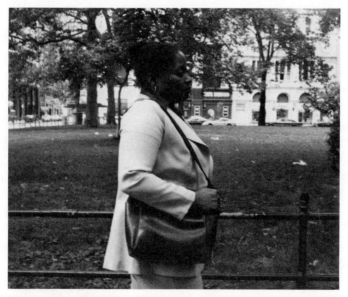

The proper technique. The bag is held secure, with the flap facing the body. The grip is not so tight that it will attract a mugger's attention.

put something where it won't be found by an experienced criminal. One thing that may help is a money belt. These can still be purchased in some clothing stores and will usually hold from 5 to 15 dollars. Another suggestion is to keep money in more than one place. The idea is to hand over your wallet and to hope that the thief won't search any further. This often works but it does involve some risk. The mugger may become angry if he goes through your pockets and finds out that he has been tricked.

A variation of this plan is to keep a dime taped to your clothing. This way even if your wallet and bills are taken, you can still get to a payphone and call for help. Another precaution is to photostat the important cards you have in your wallet. These duplicate copies should be left at home. They cannot be used, but they will be helpful if you are robbed and have to replace the originals.

These are important points, but we are getting away from the topic of this section: "When is crime more likely to occur?" My answer to that question is that you are more vulnerable when you are alone, when you are on streets that aren't busy, and when you are carrying a pocketbook that is easy to grab.

WHAT WE DO WRONG TO ATTRACT A MUGGER

A professional mugger usually knows when a person is carrying a large amount of money. He finds out not by noticing how a person is dressed but by noticing how the person is acting. There are certain signals that we can give to a mugger that let him know that we have more money than usual.

What are the clues that betray us? One is that when we have a large sum of money, we tend to look nervously about to make sure that we are not being followed. Another clue is that when our wallet is full, we keep patting it to make sure that it is still there. Women with a lot of money in their pocketbook will tend to clutch it very tight. All of these signs are noticed by the experienced mugger.

Muggers who study their victims will be attracted to the persons who receive their mail and head straight to the bank. Other likely targets are people who hurry to the bank as soon as they get out of work. These are probably people who have been paid and who are rushing to cash their checks.

There may be times when you actually show your money to a potential mugger. This can be avoided by careful planning. For example, when you go to the supermarket, try to know in advance how much you are going to spend. Take out enough money to cover your bill and keep this cash in one of your pockets. When it comes time to pay, you can use this money instead of opening your wallet or purse in front of everyone on line.

It is also a good idea not to discuss any personal plans while you are on line. If someone overhears that you are due to go on vacation, they can plan to rob you in two different ways: (1) They can follow you home and plot a burglary for the time when you will be away. (2) They can watch you for the next few days, knowing that you will soon be withdrawing cash to make your trip.

WHAT YOU SHOULD DO IF YOU SUSPECT DANGER

When I interview victims, I sometimes hear that they were attacked from behind—that they never heard the mugger coming. When this happens, there is no chance to use preventive self-protection. But other times victims get advance warnings. Some of these signals come from within. They may be a quick heart beat, a sick feeling in the stomach, or a sudden chill. All of these symptoms are the body's way of reacting to potential danger. I call this reaction the "sixth sense."

Everyone has this extra sense, but not everyone recognizes its signal and not many people heed its warning. For example, suppose you think you are being watched by a person who seems to be dangerous. Your heart may start to beat faster. You may suddenly become short of breath. Your body is telling you that you are in danger, but how will you react? Will you run? Will you yell for help? Will you decide to do nothing?

From experience I can tell you that most people would decide to do nothing. Why? Because they are not willing to trust their sixth sense. They are afraid that if they react and their intuition is wrong they will look foolish. This is true, but suppose they don't react and their intuition was right.

If you suspect danger, the first thing to do is ask yourself what is available. The answer to that question will depend on the situation. But one response that is almost always appropriate is calling for help. The best way to do this is to yell. This lets everyone know that you are in trouble and it warns the mugger that he cannot commit the crime without being noticed.

People who have trouble yelling have sometimes been advised to

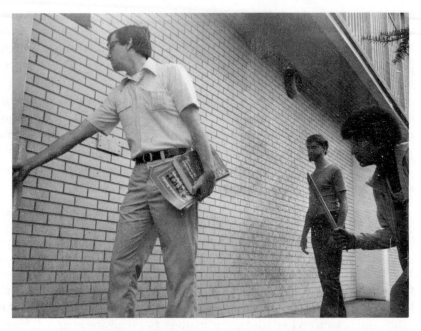

The victim is stalked by two would-be attackers.

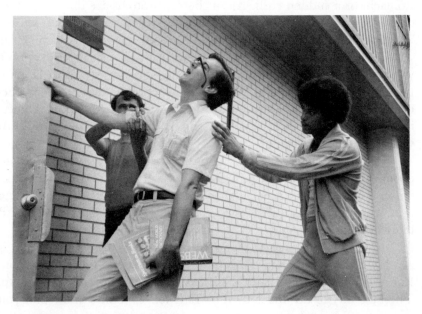

Unaware of the impending danger, the victim is struck from behind and rendered helpless.

carry whistles. The whistle is a good attention getter, but it may not be effective unless people recognize that it is a call for help. Another drawback to the whistle is that it can be used against you. An irate or panic-stricken mugger can shove it down your mouth and cause you to choke. For this reason, a few communities in New Jersey have experimented with a hand-held noisemaker. This is a safer device, but it will only get you help if people understand why it is being used.

CRIME PREVENTION IN THE DANGER ZONES

What areas do you consider dangerous in your own neighborhood or city? Do you avoid walking through the park at night? Are there corners that you stay away from because they are hangouts for local gangs? Do you bypass certain streets or public places because they have a reputation for crime? If so, you would consider these places *danger zones*. But if you are new in the neighborhood, you will not be aware of these trouble spots. In this case, you should visit your local police station to find out where you are most likely to be victimized.

In addition to the neighborhood danger zones, there are other hazardous areas that we often overlook. For example, many muggings occur on our streets, in parking lots, on elevators, in the laundry room, or at the front door of our own homes. We cannot avoid these places; they are part of our everyday life. We can approach them, however, with a greater awareness. The rest of this section will suggest a few precautions that should become part of our daily routine.

Precautions to be Taken on the Street

When you are on the street, you have to be a little bit cautious. I don't suggest that you study each person who passes or that you turn around to make sure that you're not being followed. If you did this, you would live in constant fear. Not only that, your behavior would be likely to attract a mugger. What I do recommend is that you keep casually aware of your surroundings—as you might do if you were driving. When you are in your car, you may be listening to the radio and talking to a friend. But you still know what is happening on the street. If somebody darts out from behind a car, you suddenly stop listening, stop talking, and step on the brake. This is an automatic reaction. The same type of a response may be necessary when you are a pedestrian. You may be walking along, enjoying the breeze, and thinking about the day at work, but you also must notice what is happening on the street. If something arouses your sixth sense, you must immediately step on the brake and say to yourself, "What do I have available?"

A tip I learned as a student driver may help you in practicing preventive self-protection. When I was first learning to drive, my father told me to watch for little feet behind parked cars. If I saw a pair of feet, I wouldn't be surprised to see a child run out into the middle of the street. This technique gave me a few seconds advance warning. The same type of watchfulness may help you detect a concealed mugger. His feet may be visible from behind a parked car, from the inside of a doorway, or from the edge of an alley.

If you are lucky enough to recognize a potential mugger, you should immediately ask yourself "What do I have available?" If the person is following you, what you have available is a way of testing him. Cross the street and walk a half a block, and—if you are still being followed—cross the street again. If the person behind you crosses the street both times, you know that you are in trouble.

What do you now have available? A good source of help may be a nearby store where you can call the police. If there are no stores around or if they are all closed, another alternative would be a sidewalk payphone. You could use this to call for help and, if the phone were enclosed in a booth, the booth would provide you with protection. With the door shut and your body leaning against it, the door is difficult to open from the outside. To get into the booth, the mugger will have to break the glass and risk being injured and attracting attention.

Of course, the payphone will not help you unless you have change. This is why I recommend that you always carry a dime. Preferably the dime should be taped to your clothes so it is only used for an emergency.

Another source of help could be a fire alarm box. People hesitate to use this because there is a penalty for sounding a false alarm. But it is better to pay a fine than to risk an encounter with a mugger.

Assuming that you cannot get to a phone or a fire alarm, you

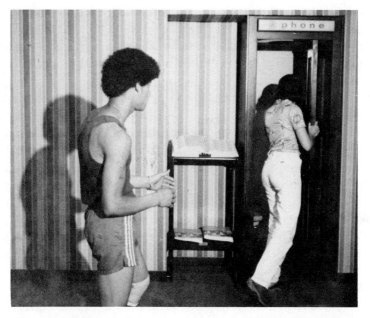

If you are being pursued by a mugger, you may find refuge in a nearby phone booth.

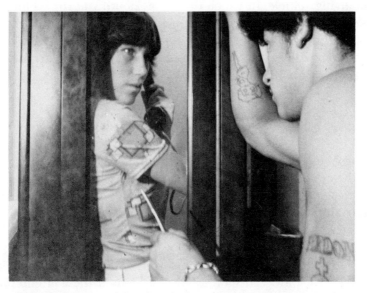

Once inside the phone booth, lean against the door so the mugger can't get in. If you have a dime, call the police.

may find safety in the middle of the street. The mugger is not likely to attack you in the midst of traffic. There is a possibility that you can escape in a passing taxi or car. But the car may be another source of danger—especially if it is driven by an accomplice of the mugger.

While you are in the street, you should not be silent. Yelling for help may get you assistance and it may scare off the would-be assailant.

Muggers do not always travel on foot. Nor do they always seem threatening. A would-be mugger in a car may stop near a pedestrian and ask for directions. As the person on foot approaches the car, the driver may open the door and pull him into the vehicle. This technique has been used for robbing, kidnapping, and for taking hostages in cases of international terrorism.

The person who approaches the car is also risking other danger and embarrassment. Predators have thrown acid or urine through a car window at an unsuspecting victim. Exhibitionists have lured people to the edge of a car and have then exposed themselves.

If someone in a car stops and asks for help, there is no reason not to cooperate. But remember to keep your distance. Do not step off the sidewalk.

If you are in the street, and you are being pursued by a person in a moving vehicle, in which direction should you run? The answer is that you shouldn't run in the same direction as the car because you can't outrun it. Your best chance is to run in the opposite direction. The driver will have to stop the vehicle and turn it around. This may give you time to get away.

Precautions to be Taken in Your Car

You probably feel secure when you are in your car, but there are two ways that a criminal can get at you. One way is to enter the car while you are stopped at a traffic light or stop sign. To prevent this, you should always drive with your doors locked and your windows no more than half way open. While you are stopped, your car should remain in gear.

If somebody tries to break into your vehicle, press down on the horn and drive away as soon as you can. Under these circumstances, you may have to drive through a red light. This is all right provided that there is no cross traffic going through the intersection.

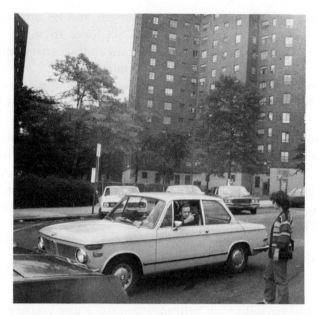

Be careful not to approach a car. If you are asked for directions, give them from the curb.

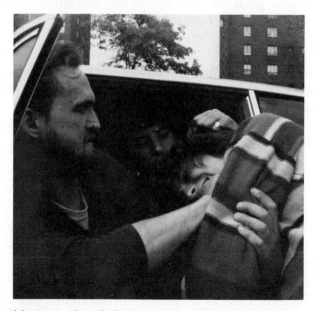

In this case, the victim is within range of the driver and passenger. She is dragged into the car and is liable to be abducted and abused.

Do not invite hitch-hikers into your car and be cautious when you are approached by pedestrians. Do not leave anything valuable where it can be seen from the street or from another car. A wallet left out on the seat may attract unwelcome company.

The other way that you can be vulnerable when you are in your car is to be followed by a criminal in another vehicle. This may escape your detection. To avoid being surprised, you should always check your rear view mirror before leaving the car. If you suspect that someone is waiting for you, do not get out. Either stay in the car with the doors locked or drive away. If you choose the second course of action and the car follows you, keep driving until you find a place where you can get help. A police station or a fire house are the most likely sources.

If you live in a private home, you may be in your own driveway before you realize that you are in danger. When this happens, the criminal can prevent you from leaving. He can either park on the street and block the exit of the driveway or he can pull into the driveway and park directly behind you. Either way you are trapped. The only thing you can do is to remain in the car with the doors locked. Hit your horn continuously so you can attract a neighbor's attention. The neighbor may call for help and the sound of your horn may scare off the attacker.

Thus, there are two danger zones when you are in your car. One is the stop light and the other is your destination. Special care must be exercised in both of these places. Whenever possible know your route in advance. Select main thoroughfares in preference to poorly lit side streets. If you get lost, do not stop a pedestrian for directions. Keep driving until you find a gas station or a policeman.

Precautions to be Taken in a Parking Lot

While street crime is more common in the city, crime in a parking lot has become a significant problem in the suburbs—especially in the parking lots of the huge shopping centers. These areas are spacious and are difficult to patrol. The mugger can use the rows of cars to conceal himself. He knows that the patrons of the shopping center are likely to be carrying large amounts of money. He will have a chance to get this money when the shoppers return to their cars and stop to open the door.

If you are visiting a shopping center, the best safety precaution is to go there with a friend. As always, you are less likely to be mugged if you are not alone. When you park your car, make sure that the doors are locked. Muggers will sometimes hide inside a car and wait for the driver to return.

At night time, always try to park near a flood light, so the area around your car will not be dark. The flood light will also serve as a landmark, which will help you to locate your car quickly. If you can walk directly to the car, you are safer than if you have to wander around the lot.

When you return to your car, try to have your key ready before you get to the door. Check inside and around the car before stopping. If the area appears to be clear, get into the car, lock the doors, and *then* arrange your packages. Do not bother with what you have bought until all the doors are safely locked.

Sometimes people will return to their car to drop off a few packages before they finish shopping. These packages should be placed inside the trunk. If they are left on a seat, they may be spotted by a thief who will break into the car to get them. When this happens, the shoppers not only lose their belongings but they risk injury if they come back to the car while the crime is in progress.

Another danger in the parking lot are the motorized purse snatchers. These people travel in groups of two or more per car. As they drive past a victim, one of the passengers reaches out and snatches her bag. The car speeds off before the victim can summon help. One way to guard against this crime is to carry your pocketbook between your packages and your body. This will make it more difficult to grab.

While parking facilities have attracted the most attention, shopping centers have had trouble in other areas. Recently several women have been molested by con artists who have posed as store detectives. In this case, the bogus detective accuses the woman of having taken goods off the shelves and having hidden them in her clothes. He takes the woman to a private room where he partially undresses her while pretending to search for stolen merchandise. Self-protection here not only requires a check of the security officer's identification but a demand to see the store manager. The woman should only agree to be searched by a female police officer. Male personnel are not permitted to make an internal search of a female suspect.

Precautions on the Subway

Over 15 million Americans live in cities that have subways. Many more people commute to work in these cities and still others visit them as tourists. Thus there are enough potential subway users to warrant our including the subways in our list of danger zones.

Like crime on the street, subway crime varies with the hour. Most pickpocketing and purse snatching takes place during the rush hour. The more desperate crimes, such as mugging and assault, occur after the business day when subway traffic is lightest.

When you board a train during these hours, avoid getting in a car that does not have many people. Once you are on the train, if you feel that you are being watched, get up and change cars. If you do this and you are followed, look for a motorman, conductor, or a transit patrolman. The conductor can use his intercom to call the next station for help. Being near a person in uniform may be all the protection you need.

Another alternative is to stand near the door. When the subway pulls into the station wait for the door to open and partially close. Then get off the train. The door should close behind you before the would-be mugger can follow you onto the platform. But remember your predicament may grow worse if the platform is isolated and the mugger is able to get off the train.

Precautions in Apartment Buildings

Mugging is not limited to the street or the outdoors; many people are victimized in their own homes or apartment buildings. In recent years this type of crime has doubled. One reason for its increase is that the mugger who strikes indoors is not likely to have many witnesses.

The danger zones in an apartment building fit one general description. They are places that can be frequented by all the tenants, but at any particular time there is a good chance that these places will be empty. Four such locations are the elevator, the laundry room, the mail room, and the staircase. These places all require extra precautions.

The person who robs on the elevator may operate in a few

different ways. He may wait in a corner of the elevator for the unsuspecting victim to enter. Or he may board the elevator at the same
time or immediately after the victim. In this case, the mugger may
push a button for one of the lower floors. When the elevator stops,
the mugger is joined by an accomplice who helps him commit the
crime. Another technique is for the mugger to get off the elevator
one floor ahead of his victim. When the mugger exits, the passenger
who is left behind quite probably feels relieved. This person may
have suspected danger and may now feel that he is safe. But while the
elevator is traveling to the next floor, the mugger is quickly running
up the steps. Imagine the terror of the victim when the elevator door
opens and he is confronted by the mugger.

Not all of the elevator techniques belong to the muggers. There
are a few rules that you can follow that may keep you from becoming
a victim. The first thing to remember is that you shouldn't get on an
elevator if you are the least bit suspicious. Don't be embarrassed
about waiting in the lobby. If someone asks you if you are going up,
you can tell them that you are waiting for a friend.

Many people get on an elevator without looking. This is especially true if they hear the elevator door closing and they don't want
to wait for the elevator to return. In this case, what they do is yell
"hold the door" and then they rush to get inside before the door
closes. Once the door is shut, the passenger is trapped. If there is a
mugger inside the car, there is no means of immediate escape.

When you ride on an elevator with other people, try to stand
sideways close to the door. In case of an emergency, you will be able
to make a fast exit. If you feel that you are going to be mugged, press
several buttons ahead of your floor. When the elevator makes its first
stop, try to get off. At this point, you may be detained or it is possible
that the crime may already be in progress. You must then ask yourself two questions: "Am I likely to be hurt as well as robbed?" and
"If I want to resist, what do I have available?" Many answers to the
second question will be presented to you in the next chapter. One
thing that you do have available is the ability to attract attention
and, possibly, to get help. While the elevator is traveling from floor
to floor, any screams for assistance will barely be heard. This is especially true if people have their doors shut and their radios or TVs
playing. But since you have pressed several buttons, the elevator
door will keep opening. When it does, your screams should be heard
by everyone on the floor.

To get the best results, I suggest that you yell "help, fire" instead of "help, police." When people hear the word "police," they may feel that the problem belongs to someone else and that they are increasing their own risk if they react. But the word "fire" suggests a danger that threatens everyone. People are likely to come out of their apartments if they think that their safety may be jeopardized. What they can do to help will be explained later in the chapter.

The laundry room is a different type of danger zone. It is usually far removed from all of the apartments. While a ride in an elevator takes just a minute, a trip to the laundry room may last for an hour. If during this time a criminal appears, the victim may be robbed, beaten, or sexually molested without anyone hearing a call for help.

When you want to use the laundry room, your best protection is the company of a friend. This will make the time go faster and will make you less vulnerable to attacks. Do not always rely on the same friend. If this person is sick or on vacation, you will have no one to take his or her place. A better idea is to make up a list of when other tenants do their laundry and to try to remember the times when the laundry room is busy. This way if your "buddy" is not available, you can do your laundry at a time when the room is occupied.

For extra protection, it is a good idea to let a neighbor know when you are going to do your laundry and when you expect to come back. If you do not return on schedule, the neighbor should call the superintendent, who should either check the laundry room or notify the police.

This second precaution will not prevent the crime from happening. It is a means of getting you help if you are injured by a criminal and unable to get out of the laundry room.

Mugging in the mail room is sometimes the result of one simple mistake. When you go to the mail box, you should remove your mail and return to your apartment. What most people do wrong is stop to sort through the envelopes to look for a letter or a check. If they are really anxious, they will open an envelope and study its contents. When this happens, people are not paying attention to their surroundings. Also, they are convincing the mugger that the envelope contains something valuable.

Some people will walk upstairs any time the elevator is not on the main floor waiting for them. This is good exercise, but the staircase can be a place of concealment for the mugger. For this reason, you may prefer to use the steps only when the elevator is not working.

When you do use the staircase, it is a good idea to have your eyes fixed one storey ahead of you. If you notice someone you don't recognize, get off the steps and ring a neighbor's doorbell.

Preventive self-protection in the apartment house depends on two things: your own use of caution and the cooperation of your neighbors. If you don't know the people who live around you, I suggest that you introduce yourself and that you invite them to call you if they should ever need your help. Once you give them your phone number, they are likely to give you their number in return. It is a good idea to keep this close to your phone so in case of an emergency there is someone nearby that you can call.

Precautions in Your Home or Apartment

There are several ways in which a criminal may gain access to your place of residence: He may follow you in off the street; he may enter through a door that you've left open; he may ring your doorbell and persuade you to let him in; he may ring your doorbell and force his way in; or he may break in through a door or a window in order to commit a burglary. Once the criminal is inside, he is extremely dangerous. If you are in the house with him, your objective should be to get to the door and to get out. If this is not possible, it may be advisable for you to use force.

There are two precautions you can take to avoid being followed into your house or apartment. Before you get to the door, try to notice if anyone is lurking in the area. If you are fortunate enough to see someone, do not open the door. Go right to a neighbor's house and ring the doorbell. This is another instance where it is important for you to trust your sixth sense.

The other safety technique is to have your key out before you get to the door. This way it will be a matter of seconds before the door is unlocked and you are safely into your home. The alternative is to fumble through your pockets as you look for the key. While you are doing this, you are losing valuable seconds and the mugger may be approaching.

People in apartment houses sometimes leave their doors open for muggers when it is time to take out the garbage. They do this because it is too much bother to shut the door behind them and to have to unlock it on the way back. While they are at the incinerator, the mugger may slip into their apartment and wait for their return. I have three rules that I recommend for this situation. (1) Don't leave your door open. A door that is not shut is an invitation to the criminal. (2) As you leave your apartment, yell inside "I'll be back in just a minute." Make a habit of doing this even if you live by yourself or if no one is home. You are less likely to be mugged if the criminal thinks that there is someone inside waiting for you. (3) Do not take out the garbage if you are not fully dressed. This may seem obvious, but many women have been molested because they went to the incinerator wearing just a nightgown.

Muggers may come to your door pretending to be salesmen, census takers, or even policemen. The important thing to remember is not to open your door for anyone you don't know. If the person outside claims to be on official business, ask him to slip his identification underneath the door. Policemen should be able to show you a shield and an identification card. If you do not see these objects, do not open the door. A door-to-door salesperson should not be permitted to enter until you find out his name and the name of his company. Once you have this information, tell the salesperson that you will call his company to confirm that he is employed there. If the salesperson is legitimate, he may wait for your return. If he is not, he may leave as soon as you go to make the phone call.

However, this means of verification is anticipated by some criminals. When you ask for their employer's phone number, they will give you the number of a cohort who is expecting just such a call. When the accomplice answers the phone, he uses the company name that his partner has given you. He assures you that the man outside your door is an employee of the company. On this basis, you let the man come in and, as a result, you may be beaten and robbed.

The best way to guard against this deception is to check the number that the salesperson has given you against the number that is listed in the phone book. If the two numbers match, the salesperson might be legitimate. But as an extra precaution you should still call the company and make sure that they employ a person of that name and description. If they don't, you know that the salesperson is a fraud and you should notify the police.

A means of gaining entry that is popular in the suburbs is the false request for assistance. In this situation, the mugger comes to the door and announces that his companion has just had a serious accident. The mugger may want to come in to get water or bandages for his injured friend. But this is not the time to comply with a stranger's request. What you can do is offer to help by phoning the police or phoning an ambulance. If the person is sincere, they will thank you for your efforts.

Apartment dwellers are probably familiar with a type of entry that is called the "push-in." The mugger who uses this technique may ring the doorbell and wait for the door to be partially opened. As soon as there is an entry way just a few inches wide, the mugger will get his foot in the door and will force his way in.

Your best defense against this type of push-in is to keep your door closed. You should have a peephole that will allow you to recognize a caller while your door is still shut. Peepholes are not expensive and are not difficult to install. You can find them at most any hardware store.

Another type of push-in occurs when the mugger is lurking in a hallway. He waits for a tenant to get off the elevator or to come up the steps. As the tenant gets to his door, the mugger quietly approaches. Once the door is open, the tenant is shoved inside and the mugger follows him in.

This type of push-in is demonstrated in the photographs. An aunt of mine, age 90, has prepared for this type of crime by keeping a club next to her door. Theoretically, if she were forced back into her apartment, she would pick up the club and defend herself. A less drastic means of protection just requires that you make a habit of being observant. When the elevator gets to your floor, look in both directions before you get off. If you notice someone whom you don't recognize, stay on the elevator.

While this is a book about mugging, it is not inappropriate to have a brief discussion about burglary. The burglar will usually try to break into your home while you are away. However, if he enters your home and finds you inside—or if you return to your home and surprise him—you may be in grave danger. For this reason, I consider the prevention of burglary an important part of preventive self-protection.

Reducing the chance of burglary is a two-step process. One precaution is obvious; you should secure all means of entry to your home. This would include locking all doors and shutting all windows. Frank Duggan, a former burglar who is now part of my staff (see the interview in Chapter 9), told me that he could enter most suburban homes through an open bathroom window. Suburbanites would leave this window open to air out the bathroom and would

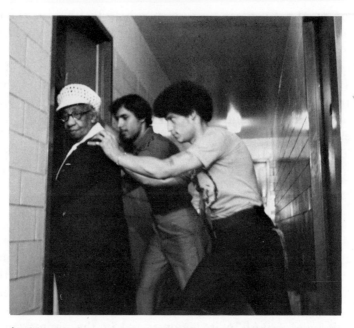

As this elderly tenant opens her door, she is shoved into her apartment.

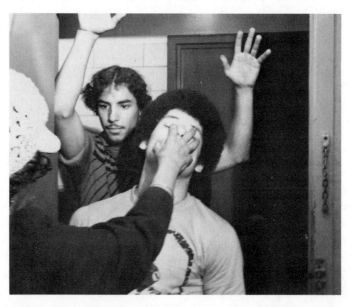

Before the muggers can follow her in, she turns and jabs one of them in the eyes.

forget about it when it was time to leave the house. The lesson is that when you are going out you should be sure to check the windows as well as the door.

The second part of burglary prevention is concealing the fact that no one is home. Many authorities suggest that you turn on a light when you are going out. Another deception that is even more convincing is to turn on your radio. If you leave for a few days, arrange to have a neighbor pick up your mail. A full mail box is a sure sign that the family is away.

When you return home, notice the doors and windows before you enter. If something seems to have changed, do not go in. Stop at a neighbor's home and phone the police.

The danger of encountering someone in your own home is demonstrated by the fact that the penalty for committing burglary is almost always severe. All types of burglarizing are considered felonies. In most states, people are not required to retreat from anyone who unlawfully enters their home. The would-be victims may use force to protect their belongings and their family. However, if you or your family are in the house at the same time as a burglar, it is a good idea to retreat if you have the opportunity.

AVOIDING DANGER AT THE SCENE OF A CRIME

My lecture on prevention is often interrupted by the question, "Officer Griffith, I did everything you said, but I still got mugged. What did I do wrong?" The answer may be "Nothing." There are some crimes that cannot be avoided. Sometimes a mugger spots his victim minutes before the victim sees the mugger. Sometimes the victim never sees the mugger at all. But the fact that some crimes are unavoidable should not discourage you from taking precautions. You should recognize, however, that while precautions reduce the likelihood of crime, they cannot eliminate it.

Preventive self-protection does not end when you are confronted by a mugger. Some would-be victims have been able to talk themselves out of being robbed—for example, a man who was approached in a parking lot pretended to be a mugger himself and berated his would-be attacker for moving in on his territory. A woman who was faced with a group of teens pretended to know one of the boys' mothers. By doing this, she convinced the boys that if they harmed her, word would get back to their parents. As a result, they left her alone. An elderly woman who was on the verge of being mugged invited her assailants to rape her. The young men were so upset by the thought of having sex with their elderly victim that they walked away in disgust. These were unique and imaginative responses to crime. They may not work in every situation.

If you are approached by a mugger, you should still think about prevention. But now prevention means avoiding injury. This can usually be accomplished in two ways: by cooperating with the mugger and by remaining calm so that you don't panic him. Some people may disagree with the first portion of this advice. They feel that they have worked hard for what they own and they are not going to give it up without a fight. This may be your reaction. If it is, I respect your feelings, but I would like you to consider another point of view. We have all read about people who have lost their lives or have been seriously injured when they fought to protect their belongings. These people were courageous, but did they make the right decision? To me, safety should come first. In every lecture, I remind the members of the audience that their wallet or purse may contain their life savings but it does not contain their life. I recommend that people never fight to protect their property.

Cooperating with the mugger may mean giving up your money and giving it up fast. Many of the muggers that I interviewed explained that they struck their victims because they did not hand over their belongings quickly enough. In these cases, a slow response was considered the same as resistance.

We all have a tendency to hang onto what we own. A woman who has her pocketbook snatched may instinctively hold onto the strap and try to pull it back. This may result in a brief tug of war, which may end with the mugger striking or even knifing the victim. Many women have been injured in this way. Their stories are particularly tragic when you realize that most of them had no intention of offering resistance. They just did what came naturally.

If your pocketbook is ever snatched, the safest response is to just let go. Since this is not a natural reaction, it may require some practice. If you drill at home, let someone in your family come up behind you and take your bag without warning. Do this several times until you are convinced that you would act the same way if your purse were snatched on the street. Before leaving the subject, let me tell you two stories about women who had their pocketbooks taken. In the first story, a woman was standing on a subway platform. A train that was not hers pulled into the station and opened its doors for a few seconds. Just as the doors were about to close, a person on the train reached out of the window and grabbed her bag. While the purse snatcher had her pocketbook, the woman was still holding onto the strap. The train started to move and before the woman could let go, she was dragged onto the tracks and killed.

Compare this story with the experience of Abbie Jean Brownell, the director of the Active Retirement Center at Pace University in New York. I referred to Ms. Brownell in the first chapter when I mentioned the woman who said she was glad that her pocketbook had been stolen. Ms. Brownell was glad because she had not resisted and she had not gotten hurt. I think you will find her own words very instructive.

Dear Grif:

Your instructions on self-defense to our group of Active Retirement Center members turned out to be very helpful to me personally. You'll be interested to know that I was accosted a couple of months ago by a man who demanded my handbag; following your instructions, I handed it over without a word and was not hurt at all. I called the police, of course, and they were very much impressed and pleased that no damage was done except the loss of the handbag, and that I was able to give them a good description of the thief. I told them about your self-defense seminars and they thought the seminars were a wonderful idea. Thank you for your very good advice.

Sincerely,

ABBIE JEAN BROWNELL

Cooperating with the mugger will usually keep him from becoming violent. Another way to prevent violence is by staying calm. Remember in Chapter 2 I said that many muggers are as scared as their victims. When this is the case, a panicky victim may cause the mugger to use force.

Remaining calm is a difficult task. After all, the mugger is trying to frighten you to get you to cooperate. You know that you are about to lose your valuables and there is some chance that you may be injured. How then can you keep from being afraid?

It is probably impossible to eliminate all fear. But you can control it to some extent by practicing. A drill of a minute a day at home will help you master techniques that will give you confidence. The drill will also get you accustomed to the idea of being mugged so that if you are ever approached on the street it will be less of a shock.

If it is important to retain your composure when you are confronted by a mugger who appears to be unarmed, it is even more important to remain calm when a mugger has a knife at your throat or a gun at your back. In this situation, the slightest yell may cause the mugger to use the knife or to pull the trigger. The response that I recommend here is to speak to the mugger very softly in a voice that is almost inaudible. You may say to him "Would you please take my money but leave my identification!" Your request should accomplish a few things: (1) You have indicated to the mugger that you are not going to resist. You have told him that it is OK if he takes your money. (2) By talking softly, you may have diverted the mugger's attention. He has to strain to hear what you are saying. This may distract him so he is not thinking about using his weapon. He may also be distracted if he stops to think about your request. Should he keep your papers or should he let you have them? (3) The third thing that you may accomplish is that you may set the tone for the rest of the crime. Your request shows that you are thinking logically and that you have control of your emotions. There is a good chance that the mugger may respond in the same way. Of course, you cannot be entirely sure of the mugger's reaction. If he does start to use his weapon, you will have to use one of the techniques in Chapter 4.

There is another type of behavior that may also panic the mugger. He may become violent if he thinks you are trying hard to study his features so you can describe him to the police. What I suggest is that you casually observe the mugger and try to remember a few characteristics: his race, his approximate age and size, and any identifying scars or marks. Do not pay much attention to clothing worn on the upper body since this can be changed. (For example, some muggers wear reversible jackets and turn them inside out after they leave the scene of a crime.) If you are trying to remember what the mugger is wearing, concentrate on his pants and shoes. It is not likely that he will change them until the end of the day.

When the mugger leaves, notice the direction in which he is heading. If he escapes by car, try to remember the license number and, if possible, the make of the car. From experience, I have found that youthful victims are very good at identifying cars.

If you have a vision problem, you can turn this to your advantage. It is not a bad idea to let the mugger know that you are blind, or almost blind, and cannot identify him.

There is another reason for stressing your handicap. Criminals have a low regard for anyone who victimizes a blind person or a person who is crippled. If a mugger is arrested for such a crime and sent to prison, he can expect harsh treatment from the prison inmates. This is a strong deterrent. As a result, many muggers will not rob a person who is disabled.

Before moving to the next section, I will mention one other technique that does not involve force. This idea was recommended to me by Pete Shivers, a former mugger who is on my staff. His suggestion is that the victim pretend to have a heart attack. Pete is not aware of anyone who has tried this, but he is confident that it would work.

If the mugger believes that his victim may be dying, he will want to leave the scene as quickly as he can. Otherwise, there is a possibility that the mugger will be apprehended and charged with homicide. This is a much more serious crime than the mugger intended. Rather than stay and face the consequences, he will probably flee.

Another advantage to this approach is that the mugger is not likely to strike a victim who appears to be dying. Thus, in a sense, the victim is "playing possum" so the predator will leave him alone.

I can see the merits of this idea, but I would hesitate to encourage its use. The average person may find it difficult to feign a heart attack. If the mugger is not convinced, the victim may be in serious danger.

WHAT YOU CAN DO TO HELP

Prevention is most effective when everyone in the community participates. Too often we think that the police are the only ones responsible for our safety. When a crime is committed and the offender is not caught, we blame the police for not giving us satisfactory protection. But we don't consider what we can do to protect ourselves.

This section will suggest how you can help to keep your neighborhood safe. There is no risk involved. You do not have to do the job of the police or take the law in your own hands. All that is needed is a concern for the welfare of the people who live around you. In other words, you will have to be a good neighbor.

Being a good neighbor when you are the victim of a crime means reporting that crime to the police and trying to describe or identify the criminal. Unfortunately, many crimes are not reported because the victims fear retribution or they feel that the police cannot help. When you fail to report a crime, you leave the criminal free to roam the streets. His next victim may be one of your neighbors or it may be you—muggers have been known to attack the same person twice. The point is when you fail to notify the police you do a disservice to the community and yourself.

The neighborly attitude contributes to crime prevention in other ways. As you recall, the likelihood of crime decreases when people travel in pairs. For this reason, friendly neighbors have established the *buddy system*. This is an effective means of preventing crime that is especially popular with people who live by themselves. Under this system, a pair of neighbors decide that they will be responsible for each other's safety. They plan to do their shopping together so that neither one will have to walk the streets alone. They may also do their laundry at the same time. If one person goes out without the other, he tells his buddy where he is going and when he expects to be back. If the person who goes out does not return on time, it is the buddy's responsibility to check his neighbor's route and, if necessary, notify the police.

Buddies will call one another daily to make sure that their partner is all right. One pair of ladies told me they used a shade signal instead of a daily phone call. The two women lived in facing apartments. Every day at noon, they would raise their shades half way. If one of the shades did not go up on schedule, the other buddy would investigate. As a result of these periodic checks, neither partner could be sick, injured, or possibly bound and gagged for very long without the other person knowing.

In every community there are some lone individuals who have no "buddies." These people are generally senior citizens who have outlived their family and friends. If you are interested in helping a neighbor, these are the people you should contact. Call them periodically to make sure that they are all right. Arrange to take them shopping with you or to do some of their shopping for them. Your interest in these people will brighten their lives and may keep them from being the victim of a crime.

How You Can Help a Victim

When you are aware of a crime in progress there are two things you can do to help: (1) contact the police and (2) make known to the victim *and* the mugger that the police are on the way. Think back to the mugging that occurs on the elevator. The victim, suspecting danger, has pressed several buttons. The elevator stops on your floor and as the door opens you hear a call for help. What can you do?

Step one is to call the police. You should have the precinct number pasted onto your phone or tacked onto a message board that is near your phone. If you can't find the number, don't take the time to look it up or to call information. Dial the operator and ask to be connected with the local police station. If you don't have a phone, open your window and shout to the people below. Hopefully, a passer-by will find a policeman or will call the station for you.

There is another way that you can help the victim. While the elevator door is still open, partially open your door and shout to the victim, "I hear you and I'm calling the police." The sound of a neighbor's voice encourages the victim. It lets him know that he is not alone—that his call for help has not been unheeded. The news that the police are on the way should have some effect on the mugger. It is possible that he can no longer commit the crime without being caught. He may decide to get off the elevator and flee from the building.

Have you endangered yourself by confronting the mugger? It is unlikely. You can get back in your apartment and shut the door before the mugger can attack you. On the street, you have to be more cautious. If you see someone being mugged, look for a payphone or a store from which you can call the police. If no phones are available, head for the nearest corner and look in all directions for a policeman. Assuming that no policeman is around, you can try to bluff the mugger by yelling "You'd better run; here come the police." The mugger cannot see in all the directions that you can and he is likely to believe that the law is just around the corner.

This type of deception will usually be successful. However, there may be some risk involved if there is not much distance between yourself and the mugger. I would not try this method if the mugger were armed with a gun.

Community Efforts Against Crime

In some areas, being a good neighbor means joining the tenants or community association. The roles of these organizations vary. One of their important functions is known as "block watching." This activity consists of a group of adults who patrol the street in a car or on foot. The purpose of block watching is to detect a crime in progress and to radio the police. This is a successful deterrent because it increases the chance that a criminal will be caught.

Some block watchers will not wait for a crime to happen. They will stop strangers on the street and ask them where they are going and what is their business. If the answers are not satisfactory, the police may be called in for further investigation.

Often the mere existence of a neighborhood patrol is enough to discourage crime. For this reason, many organizations have posted signs indicating that an area is being watched. The sign lets the criminal know that there is an extra risk in working this neighborhood. Relating this to the elements of a crime, we can say that when an area is being watched, there is less chance of committing a crime successfully and less chance of the criminal getting out of the neighborhood without being caught.

In addition to block watching, groups of civilians (known as tenants associations) have patrolled large apartment buildings. Persons on duty have questioned anyone in the halls or lobby that they did not recognize. As a result of these actions, crime was reduced and all the tenants felt more secure.

In 1977, a teenage tenants association in the Bronx was commended by the mayor for their outstanding service during the blackout. The association helped many people and prevented the looting that took place in other parts of the city. The benefits of this type of a program are obvious. Not only does the neighborhood profit from the service of the teenagers, but the young people are given a chance to do something constructive for the community. This is a character-building experience that residents in many areas should encourage.

While there is a danger that block watchers or building watchers may turn into vigilante groups, so far the history of this activity has been good. The main problem that plagues these organizations is that after a while their members become complacent. When the organization is formed, everyone is enthusiastic. As the incidence of crime starts to decrease, the enthusiasm continues. But after a while, people become accustomed to the lower crime rate. There appears to be less need for the association and many of the members start to drop out. As the membership dwindles, more and more responsibility is heaped on a few active citizens. People develop an attitude of "Let the other guy do it." The association suffers and, eventually, the neighborhood suffers too.

Despite this drawback, crime prevention groups have been successful and have attracted the attention of the FBI. In 1975, it sponsored neighborhood crime resistance in four different areas. In Birmingham, Alabama, an organization was formed to limit the trafficking in stolen property. In DeKalb County, Georgia, the purpose of the organization was to prevent crimes against youths. In Norfolk, Virginia and Wilmington, Delaware, the target offenses were—respectively—crimes against women and crimes against the elderly. The initial reports on these ventures were good. The interest of the FBI strengthens the assumption that I made at the beginning of this section: Citizens can participate in crime prevention. Or, stated more simply, with the help of the police, we have the ability to protect ourselves.

4

Fighting for Your Life

This chapter presents most of the techniques that comprise my mini-system of self-defense. Before you read further, I would like you to examine your own feelings about using force to protect yourself. Do you think, if it were necessary, you would be able to fight back against a mugger? Many people are skeptical.

They feel that if they were confronted by a mugger they might be paralyzed by fear. Or, if they were able to control their fright, they doubt that they would be able to think fast enough to catch the mugger by surprise. (It is interesting to note that these doubts are sometimes shared by young soldiers who are taught the methods of hand-to-hand combat. The soldiers may perform the techniques flawlessly in drill, but they tend to disbelieve that they could ever use them successfully in battle.)

What are the capabilities of the average victims? Are they able to think quickly and objectively? Can they control their emotions so they are able to protect themselves from a dangerous criminal? A leading researcher in the field of victimology—Dr. Martin Symonds of the Karen Horney Institute—thinks not. He believes that most victims are not able to cope with their predicament. He attributes their lack of ability to a phenomenon that he calls "frozen fright." In a recent article, Dr. Symonds stated:

> We have found that the vast majority of people, both men and
> women, respond similarly to violent crime. The immediate response
> of an individual who meets with sudden unexpected violence is
> momentary shock and disbelief. This phase is quickly followed by a
> frozen-frightened response which seems only to permit submissive,
> compliant, and ingratiating behavior to the perceived overwhelming
> threat to life. The reaction of fear is so profound and overwhelming

that the victim feels hopeless about getting away. All hope of survival is dependent on appeasing the criminal. . . .

There are other individuals whose response to sudden unexpected violence is not frozen fright but anger. Even though their behavior is rooted in profound fright, the victims recall only being angry. They screamed, hit, or yelled. They said to the criminal: "Get the hell away. What are you doing? Leave me alone, I'll call the police." Some have attacked the criminal with their purse, their hands, or thrown things at him. What happens to the victim depends on circumstances and on the mental health of the criminal. While some back down and even run away, more often the criminal feels frustrated and angry. This results in a violent attack on the victim to beat him or her into submission and compliance. A woman said to a criminal who was robbing her store: "I'll never forget your face." He shot her in the head and blinded her.

> Dr. Martin Symonds, *"Victims of Senseless Violence,"* Psychiatric Worldview, *Vol. 1, No. 1 (Jan./March 1977). Presented by Lederle Laboratories.*

If you have read the first three chapters, you know that my outlook is more optimistic than what is expressed in the passages above. This does not mean that "frozen fright" does not exist or that it might not be your reaction if you were mugged. But I do believe that it is possible to guard against it. There may be a difference between you and the victims described by Dr. Symonds. Hopefully, by the time you have finished this book, you will have had the benefits of preparation. I believe that preparation can protect you from the paralyzing fear of frozen fright. If you are adequately prepared, you should be able to respond quickly—even if you are in the presence of a mugger.

To demonstrate the value of preparation, let us look briefly at the evolution of a policeman. He starts out—like all of us—as a civilian. But once he is in uniform we do not expect him to go into frozen fright when he is confronted by danger. We expect him to act dependably. But why should he react differently from another human being? Part of the answer can be attributed to his training.

When recruits come to the academy, they are taught how to protect themselves. As they learn how to use their strength and their weapons, they develop a confidence that stays with them when they are subjected to danger. This confidence does not eliminate fear. But it tempers fear so that, even in danger, the policeman can think objectively.

As part of their training, recruits are introduced to situations that they may have to face when they are on duty. Thus, before they go out on the streets, they have developed some experience. This experience will prevent them from being overcome by shock or surprise when they are confronted by new situations. Another advantage of considering problems ahead of time is that it gives the policeman a chance to start thinking. Thus, by the time a problem occurs, the policeman may already know what type of action is needed.

From their early training, policemen derive both confidence and experience. These are the qualities I hope to pass onto you as you read this chapter. Your confidence should come as you learn the techniques and start to believe in your ability to protect yourself. One way that you will gain experience is by reading the stories in this chapter about different mugging situations. As you become more familiar with the behavior of the mugger, you will have a better idea of how to act in his presence.

As I promised, you will soon read about the techniques that I demonstrate in my lectures. Knowing when to use these techniques is the subject of the next section.

KNOWING WHEN TO USE FORCE

Those of you who listened to Jack Benny on the radio may remember the episode when he was confronted by an armed mugger. The dialogue went something like this:

Mugger: (Threateningly) Your money or your life!
J. Benny: (Silence)
Mugger: (Impatiently) Well!
J. Benny: I'm thinking! I'm thinking!

For Jack Benny, playing the role of the penny pincher, the decision was difficult. But for you and I the choice should be easy. We would not want to jeopardize our lives to save any amount of money.

Although most people would agree with this in theory, it is not uncommon for someone to behave differently when they are actually robbed. Some people will risk their lives to protect a small amount of property. Does this seem incredible? Let us consider just one example—one that you will remember from Chapter 3.

Every year several women are injured by purse snatchers. Many of these casualties could be avoided if the women did not offer resistance. But when the women first felt their bags being yanked away, they responded by instinct. They tightened their grip on the strap and began to pull back. This usually led to a tug of war that was often terminated by the purse snatcher attacking the victim. As a result, many victims sustained injuries. These injuries were costlier—in terms of discomfort and money—than the contents of the pocketbooks that the women were trying to save.

If we had asked these people before they were attacked, "Do you think it's worth a concussion (or any type of injury) to save $10 and your driver's license?" they probably would have said "no." Why then did they risk being injured? One reason is that they were governed by the instinctive desire to hold onto their personal property. Another explanation for their noncompliance is that they did not recognize that their life was in danger.

Don't let the second mistake endanger you. Every person who tries to rob us potentially offers us the same choice that was given to Jack Benny—our money or our life. If we consider resistance in these terms, we are likely to agree with the following guideline: *Do not use force to protect personal property.*

Let me repeat what I stress in class. Your life savings may be kept in your wallet or purse, but your wallet or purse does not contain your life. If a criminal is only after your money, I strongly urge you to give it to him. Do not try to resist.

In Chapter 2, you read about the predatory mugger. This is the criminal who may not be satisfied with your money. After he has your belongings, he may continue to abuse you for any one of several reasons. He may want to scare you so you will be too terrified to identify him; he may want to disable you so you cannot prevent him from getting away, or he may want to hurt you just to satisfy his own need for physical dominance or sadistic pleasure. This type of criminal is in the minority. But if you encounter him, it is best to be prepared to use force. What I suggest here is that you give the mugger everything he demands. If after he has taken your property, he continues to abuse you, it may be time for you to retaliate. In this situation, you are not fighting to protect property, you are fighting to protect yourself.

The decision to use force can only be made by you. In making this decision, you are in the same position as the policeman who is considering whether he should use his gun. No one can tell him when he should fire. He must rely on his instinct to determine whether his life or the life of anyone else is in danger. If he feels that this is the case, then he will use his weapon.

In the same way, you must depend on your sixth sense to know if the mugger is interested in you rather than your money. If he is, his motivation may be abduction, sexual abuse, or physical violence. Where this appears to be the case, you must use one of the techniques that you are going to learn.

THREE RULES TO REMEMBER

The last section talked about the decision to use force. This is the first step in getting away from a mugger. The next step is to stop and ask yourself, "What do I have available?"

The answer to this question depends on how you are being held by the mugger, where he is most vulnerable, and where he is looking. Usually, when we think about using force, we think about using our hands or fists. But sometimes our hands are not available; they may be in the grasp of the mugger. When this is the case, we are still not helpless. There are other things we can use to get free. For example, in the next two chapters you will read about techniques that require the use of your feet, knees, elbows, fingernails, or teeth. In addition to these parts of the body, you may be carrying things that you can use to protect yourself. Good examples of these convenient weapons are the cane and the umbrella. The proper way to use these is explained later in this chapter.

Asking yourself what you have available is so important that I call it "your key to safety." If you are attacked and you remember this question—and nothing else—you still have a chance. Once you have answered this question, the next step is the actual use of force.

The next two chapters will show you several methods of using force effectively. At this point, let me mention two more rules that apply to every technique. One rule can be remembered by the acronym "KISS." The letters stand for the words "Keep It Short and

Simple." The rule tells us not to try a counterattack that requires a great amount of strength or several complex moves. In most cases, the simpler the method, the greater the likelihood of success.

Thus, as you read on, you will see that most of the methods of escape involve just two or three procedures. For example, the first technique that is shown in this chapter is the method of getting away from a mugger who has grabbed you from behind. The action I recommend is that you grab the mugger's small finger and pull it back and away from your body. As you do this, you step out of his grip and run for safety. The reason this is successful will be explained when you read about this technique. I mention it now to demonstrate its simplicity. This is an example of getting a maximum result out of a minimum of effort.

Before we discuss the final rule, let us review the steps that we have taken so far. The first step is to decide that force is necessary; the second is to ask the question "What do I have available?"; the third is to apply force in order to get away. These three steps lead us to the final step, which is to escape without getting hurt. This is the purpose of using force. The idea of fighting back is not to get revenge and not to recover your belongings. What you are trying to accomplish is to get free so you can avoid being injured. Stated another way, "The reason for using force is to escape."

This is what I consider the final rule. It is a good thing to remember as you apply the techniques. Don't try to outfight your opponent or to outmuscle him. You are not engaged in a contest of strength; you are trying to escape. Thus, while some of the techniques are designed to inflict pain, the purpose of hurting the mugger is to get him to let go or to disable him long enough so you are able to get away.

Once you *are* away, you should run toward an open and occupied area—not to an alley way where you can be trapped. And not to a deserted spot where you can be recaptured and the mugger can resume the attack without being seen. Part of getting away is yelling for help. This may discourage the mugger from chasing after you.

In this section, I have introduced three rules that are worth repeating:

1. When you decide to use force, ask yourself, "What do I have available?"
2. When you apply force, remember to keep it short and simple.

3. As you are fighting back, remember that the object of using force is to escape from the mugger without being hurt.

The fact that the victim is not trying to "win a fight" makes the whole system more believable. You, the reader, might find it hard to picture a frail senior citizen beating up a large young mugger who is carrying a weapon. But it is not too difficult to imagine the same victim doing something unexpected that hurts the mugger and gives the smaller person an opportunity to get away. This is what self-protection is all about.

Up to now, I have been talking in generalities. The remainder of this chapter will describe specific mugging situations and will recommend techniques that can be used when force is necessary. Please read slowly and go back over a paragraph when a point does not seem clear. As you finish reading about each technique, try to take time and practice it. Then go on to the next section.

RESISTING THE UNARMED MUGGER

By "unarmed mugger," I mean the criminal who attacks you without a visible weapon. It is a mistake to think that this person is not dangerous. He may have a concealed weapon or he may be working with an accomplice. The fact that he attacks the victim by surprise, and that his motives are secret, gives this mugger an advantage. Like the criminal who is armed, he should be treated with extreme care.

One Way to Get Free
When the Mugger Grabs You from Behind

When artists or photographers try to portray a mugging, they usually show the mugger behind the victim with the mugger's hand clasped over the victim's mouth. This is a common tactic for muggers for the following reasons:

1. By coming from behind, the mugger can catch his victims by surprise and can rob them without being identified.
2. The sudden appearance of a hand over the victim's face helps to intimidate the victim and makes him more likely to cooperate.

3. By covering the mouth, the mugger prevents the victim from yelling for help.
4. In this position, the victim can easily be dragged to a more secluded place.

If you are grabbed from behind and your mouth is covered, your immediate reaction may be shock. You cannot yell for help, but you do have other means of escape. Both of your hands are free. The problem is how to use them properly.

Before I suggest what you should do, let me describe two techniques that are likely to fail. There is a common tendency to grab the mugger's arm as if it were a chinning bar and to try to pull it down away from your mouth. When you attempt this, you are pitting your strength against the mugger's. In this position, the mugger has the advantage.

Another response that is not recommended is to try to punch backwards at the mugger. When you do this, your blows have little force and it is not likely that you will hit the mugger in a sensitive area.

What you should do is to notice which hand the mugger has over your mouth. If he is using his right hand, lift your right hand and grab one of his fingers (preferably the pinky or thumb). Bend the finger back as hard as you can and pull it away to the right. As the finger is yanked away from your mouth, the rest of the hand will follow.

Now you can yell for help, but more important you have hurt your attacker. The joints of the finger lock. When the finger is pulled back, the first reaction is pain and the end result can be a broken bone. If the mugger has been holding your arm or body with his other hand, the sudden pain in his finger should cause him to release his grip. This is your opportunity to escape.

Start to run and look for an open area. Avoid dead ends or alley ways, where there is a chance that you will be recaptured. With each step, remember to yell for help. By doing this, you may discourage the mugger from chasing after you.

Once you have broken free, what is the chance that you will be attacked again? There is no guarantee that the mugger won't catch you and resume the attack. But remember the three elements of a crime: the desire to commit the crime, the ability to commit the crime successfully, and the ability to escape after the crime is committed. To a great extent, you have reduced the second and third elements. The mugger has less chance for success because now he has to catch you and he knows that you can protect yourself. At the same time, there is a greater chance that he will be caught. Why? Because your screams for help may have attacted the attention of an unseen policeman.

Each technique in this chapter is followed by a short story and a series of photographs. These sequences were created especially for this book. The purpose of including them was to show you how the techniques could be used in a real-life situation. Thus, you can read about other people and develop some understanding of what it feels like to be mugged. This will allow you to be better prepared if you, yourself, are ever a victim.

To make the stories as realistic as possible, I have constructed them from events that actually happened—events that were described to me during my interviews with victims. These victims were not always aware of their available means of escape. Consequently, unlike the people in the pictures, some of these victims were seriously injured.

The victims in the pictures were not actually involved in the events depicted in the stories. The men who portray the muggers, however, were at one time convicted of similar crimes. I have used them—with their consent—to give you a better idea of what a mugging looks like. While we were taking the pictures, these ex-criminals served as both models *and* advisors. In many cases, they demonstrated exactly how a crime would be committed. Their contributions have helped to make the photographs authentic.

To see how much you have learned, read each story and put yourself in the victim's place. Ask yourself how you would have responded if you were the one who was being mugged. Then look at the photographs and cover up the captions. Can you describe what is happening in each picture? If you can, you are ready to learn the next technique.

A LIKELY STORY   Susan usually picked up her mail in the lobby and brought it directly upstairs. But on this day, she was expecting something special. She stopped in front of the mail box and thumbed through all the letters until she found the right one. Then she opened the envelope and began to study its contents. She was so engrossed that she didn't notice the man who was approaching from behind. Suddenly, she felt a tug at her left arm. Before she could yell for help, a hand was thrust over her mouth and her body was bent back. Without saying a word, her unknown attacker started to drag her back toward the stairs.

What should she do? The man had not asked her for money. He had not tried to take her pocketbook. Was he after something valuable or was he going to hurt her? Susan decided that she couldn't wait to find out. She reached up for the hand across her mouth and grabbed it by the smallest finger. She pulled it back until her mouth was free and she could hear the man grunt with pain. At this moment, the man suddenly relaxed the grip on her left arm. Susan lunged forward and ran out the door toward the street. As she saw some neighbors, she started to yell, "Help me, help me, I'm being attacked."

• • • The mail box can be a danger zone—especially at the beginning of the month when senior citizens receive their social security checks. By lingering over her mail, Susan tipped off the mugger that she was expecting something valuable. By stopping to read her mail, she let down her guard and became an easy target.

Would you have reacted in the same way? Study the picture sequence and see if you can provide your own commentary. Try to memorize this procedure before you read about the next technique.

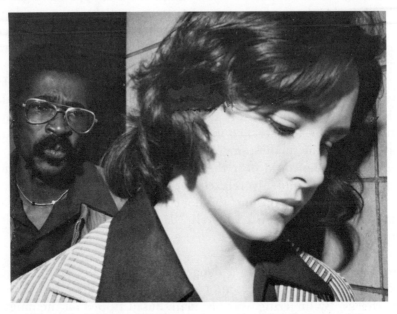

Engrossed in her mail, Susan does not notice the man who is standing behind her.

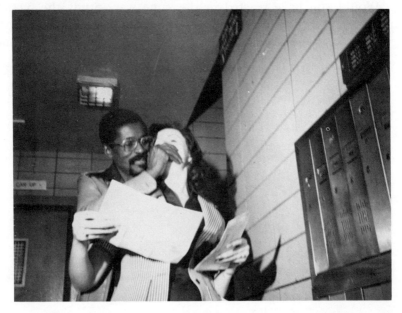

He covers her mouth, so she cannot yell for assistance.

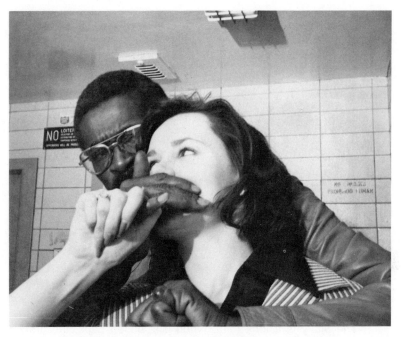

With her right hand, Susan grabs the man's pinky.

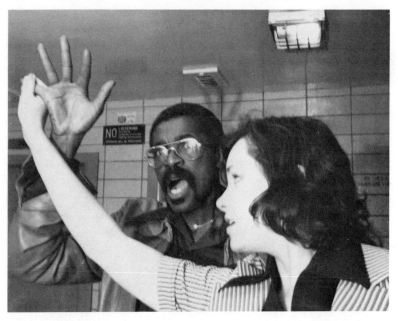

She pulls it back and draws the hand away from her face.

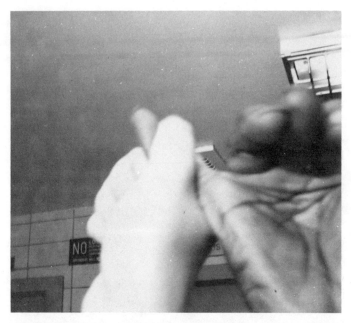

The pinky is a lock joint. When it is pulled back, the first reaction is pain and the end result can be a broken bone.

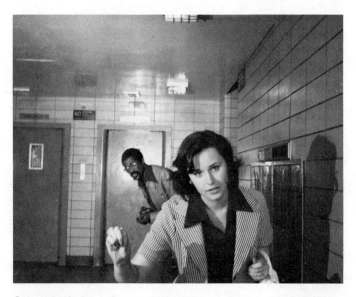

Once she is free, Susan doesn't try to recover her mail. She runs toward the street.

Eluding the Wrist Grab

When people attend my lecture for the first time, they are often skeptical. They may ask themselves two questions: "Will this really work?" and "Will this work for me?" The first question is easy for me to answer. I can refer to the many people who have used my methods successfully. To deal with the second question, I try to show that my system is easy to learn. I do this by starting my lecture with one of the easiest techniques—the escape from the wrist grab.

You can learn this technique just as if you were in my class. All you have to do is hold either arm straight out in front of you. Then bend your elbow so that your hand snaps back toward your chest. Or bring your arm straight down so it is in its normal position at your side. Do this two or three times. If a mugger had grabbed you around the wrist, one of these movements would be all you would need to escape. The secret is to see where the mugger's thumb and fingers are joined and to pull your arm from that point. The force of your arm against the mugger's thumb and fingers will always cause them to open.

A distraction will also help you when you are using this technique. What I suggest is that when you are about to break loose, you raise your free hand to the mugger's eye level and you snap your fingers. This unexpected move diverts the mugger's attention and helps you to get away.

After I demonstrate this method in class, my assistants go into the audience and grab each person by the wrist. The people use this technique to pull free and almost always succeed. The only time someone doesn't get loose is when they become overconfident and forget to look for the juncture of the fingers and thumb. The ease of this method usually convinces people that my techniques are easy to learn.

You might wonder when the wrist grab would be used. The mugger might apply this grip if he were going to pull you or if he was going to strike with a weapon that was held in his other hand. An example of the first use was told to me by a senior citizen from Flushing, New York.

She was walking down the street and didn't notice a man concealed in a doorway. As she passed the man, he seized her wrist and tried to drag her inside. Her immediate impulse was to resist. She pulled back with all her strength and started to scream. Somehow she kept herself from being pulled inside the building. Her screaming attracted several people, and the sight of the crowd frightened the mugger, who let go and ran. The woman was not struck by her attacker, but the cost of her resistance was a dislocated shoulder.

When I met this woman at one of my classes, she asked me what she had done wrong. I explained that her mistake was to pull straight back. By doing this, she was not releasing the mugger's grip. Since she was holding her ground but was not strong enough to pull the mugger toward her, all the strain of her effort was focused on her shoulder and upper arm. It was this strain that was responsible for the injury.

Compare this story with the success of someone who used the technique that you just learned. Jean Lax from the Lighthouse of the Blind was walking down the subway steps when she was struck by a weapon and her wrist was grabbed. Her resourceful escape is best explained in her own words.

Dear Liddon:

As I attempt to express our appreciation for giving such a fine self-defense seminar at the Lighthouse, there is a sad bit of irony to my thanks. . . .

The day after I appeared on the 7 and 11 o'clock news, successfully throwing off my would-be rapist, I was in reality assaulted. Coming down the subway steps about 3 P.M., I suddenly felt as if I had been slapped very hard on the rear. I turned around to find a young man wielding a knife at me. He grabbed my right arm, but I broke loose using the Griffith technique, perhaps. It happened so fast and was so very real that there was no time to think. My only response was to get away if at all possible. He tried to grab or tear my clothing, but my top was of a loose elastic and as I pulled back, he lost his grip.

Rather than feeling fear, I felt outraged that someone would attempt to violate me in this way. I stared him in the eyes and as if I were scolding a naughty child, I said, "Come on, what are you doing?" Luckily, people started coming down the stairs and he turned and ran away.

It wasn't until I was waiting for the police to arrive that I realized he had not slapped me but slashed me with his knife. The wound was only superficial, but the sight of my own blood brought home to me how much trouble I had actually been in. Perhaps he was one of the small percentage you told us about who would not hesitate to kill. It is not clear to me what his intent was, but as the sting in my backside (and the gash in my best pair of jeans) can attest, he meant business.

So in a very personal way, I thank you for being such a fine teacher. Perhaps what saved me there in the subway was the realization that although indeed I was in trouble, I was not helpless. As it turned out, I seemed to be the one in the audience for whom a crash course in self-defense was of immediate importance. . . .

Sincerely,

JEAN LAX

At this point, the alert reader will want to know "What happens if the mugger grabs your arm with both hands?" Under these circumstances, a different technique is needed. You must stop and ask yourself "What is available?" The most obvious answer is the hand that is still free. Here is the way it should be used.

First, make a fist with the hand that is being held. Then, with your free hand, reach over and grab the underneath part of your fist. (Your palm should be resting on top of your fist and your fingers should be curled underneath.) The next move is to pull your fist up and out.

When this method is tested in class, it is just as successful as the escape from the one-arm wrist grab. But not everyone is convinced. People sometimes wonder if the mugger can't stop you from using the other hand. This seems unlikely since both of the mugger's hands are clasped around your wrist.

THREE STORIES IN ONE   Donna got out of work early and started for the subway. It was a Friday afternoon and there were still hours of daylight to be enjoyed and a long weekend before it was time to go back to work. As Donna walked, her fingers strummed the iron bars of a fence. She slapped the last bar of the fence and passed a stairwell without lowering her hand. As her arm dangled in the air, it was suddenly snatched by a person standing on the steps. Although Donna jumped back in surprise, she was not yet afraid. She assumed that the person on the steps was a prankster—probably one of the young men in her office. Imagine her fear as she turned and saw a stranger clutching her arm and waving a knife in his other hand.

The stranger pulled her to the edge of the stairwell and was trying to force her to the bottom, where she could not be seen from the street. Every muscle in Donna's body fought back. As she got close to the top of the stairs, she planted her feet and leaned in the other direction. With her captured arm, she pulled straight back.

All of these efforts would probably be wasted. Not only was Donna trying to outmuscle her stronger opponent, but she was working against another disadvantage. She was pulling up while the attacker was pulling down. It would take considerable force just to stay where she was.

• • • Let us stop the story and go back to where Donna first saw the stranger. Suppose that her emotions were both fear and anger. She was scared for her life, but she was also furious at the man who was abusing her. In this state of mind, she looked at her hand and wrist as personal property—something the attacker had no right to grab. Instead of pulling back, she was determined to pull her arm away. She swung it from left to right and it snapped through the lock that was formed by the attacker's thumb and fingers. As the man let go, Donna's hand shot back so fast that it almost hit her. Stunned by her success, she paused for a second and then turned and ran.

This second story has a happy ending because the girl instinctively made the right move. She bent her arm and pulled it through the spot where the man's thumb and fingers were joined. When she got free, her first reaction was surprise. She froze for a moment just as a batter might freeze at home plate when he's hit a long ball. When the batter stops to admire his hit, he loses a step in his race to first. In the same way, when Donna stopped and said to herself "I'm free," she lost a step in her race to safety. Since her attacker was armed, the loss of a step could have been fatal.

• • • We will now take the knife away from Donna's attacker and let him put both hands around her wrist. With this hold, the man is pulling with much more force and his grip is much more secure. Donna's mood in this situation is a combination of fear and confidence. She recognizes the danger of her position, but she also knows a way out. As the man pulls harder, Donna reaches through the 'V' formed by his two arms and grabs her own fist. She lifts it up and pulls it back toward her. The move is so efficient that as Donna breaks free, the man just stops and stares. Donna has a head start as she runs toward a busy intersection.

• • • Donna's emotional state was different in each of the three stories. In the first story, she was just frightened. In the second, she was frightened and angry. In the last episode, she was still afraid but she also was confident. What would be your mood if you were attacked? Would you rely on one of these techniques? If not, what would be your alternative?

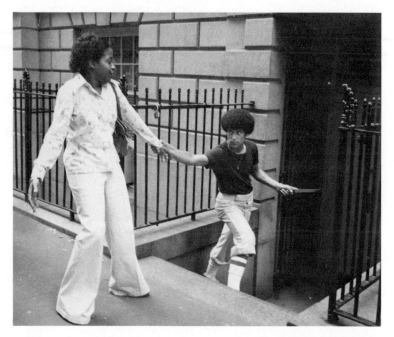

Donna is surprised by a young man standing on the steps.

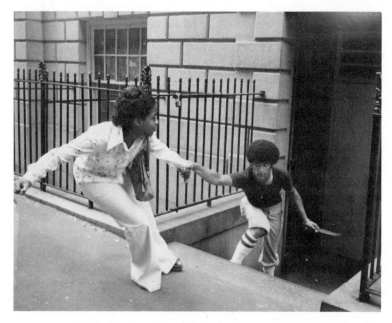

She pulls back, but is unable to get free.

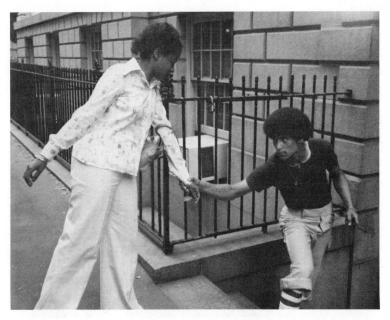

This time she looks for the place where the man's forefinger and thumb are joined.

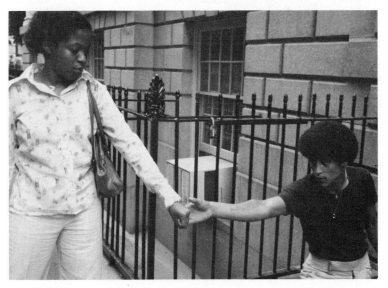

She snaps her arm through the juncture of the thumb and fingers and easily gets free.

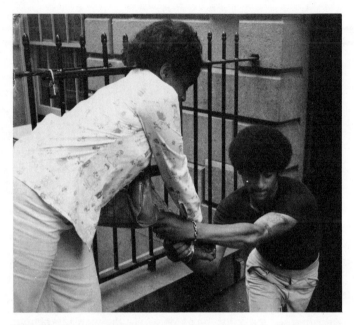

The attacker grabs Donna's wrist with both of his hands.

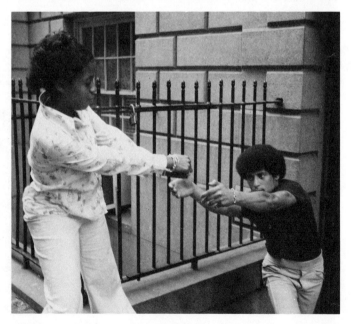

With her free hand, she reaches through the 'V' formed by the mugger's arms. She grabs her own fist and pulls it up and out of the mugger's grasp.

Escaping from the Yoke

What kind of victims do muggers prefer? Will they usually attack a child, woman, or elderly person before they will attempt to rob an adult male? Many young men believe this. They feel that the mugger will pass them by because they are more likely to offer resistance. But some muggers may disagree.

The professional mugger may prefer male victims because he feels they are likely to be carrying large sums of money. While a man may rival the mugger in strength, the criminal still has a few advantages: (1) he attacks by surprise; (2) he may have a weapon for protection; and (3) he may work with a partner who can help him if the victim starts to fight back.

One hold that is commonly applied to the male victim (although it can also be used with females) is the yoke. To get the victim in this grip, the mugger approaches from behind and locks his right arm around the victim's throat. The mugger then scoops his left hand under the victim's left armpit and with this hand he grabs his own right wrist. An experienced mugger can do this quickly. Once his two arms are joined, the hold is very difficult to break.

The mugger pulls his right arm with his left hand to tighten the grip around the victim's throat. At this point, the victim can either be choked into submission or dragged back to a secluded spot where he can be beaten and robbed.

What can the victim do to protect himself? His first move should be to turn his head to the right so he is looking over the mugger's elbow. Where the mugger's right arm is bent, there is some extra space between the arm and throat. If the victim turns his head to this spot, he shifts the pressure from his windpipe to the side of his neck. By doing this, he relieves the immediate danger of death by strangulation. (This is a very real concern. Not long ago a woman perished shortly after she was mugged on the street. She was caught in the yoke and the mugger's grip was so tight that it fractured her windpipe.)

Turning the head is a safety precaution, but it is not a means of escape. Let us see what the victim has available to break loose. The victim's right arm is free and may be used to pull down the mugger's right elbow. This will not release the grip, but it will give the victim extra breathing room.

The left arm of the person being attacked is only partially free. Its movement is impeded by the position of the mugger's left arm beneath the victim's armpit. The victim cannot use his left hand to separate the mugger's arms at the place where they are joined. But he can use his left hand to disable the mugger. There are two ways that this can be accomplished.

The victim can extend his left thumb and jab it back into the mugger's left eye. (I have previously suggested that the victim turn his head to the right to avoid strangulation. But when he is going for the assailant's eyes, the victim should twist his head to the left to be sure his thumb is traveling in the right direction.) If the mugger is struck in the eye, the pain may be severe enough to cause him to release the grip. If the thumb misses the eye or if the mugger persists in the hold, a second method can be employed.

To use this method, the victim pivots to the right so that his body is now at a slight angle to the mugger. Before, the victim's back was covering the mugger's entire body. Now that the victim has turned, a portion of the mugger's body is exposed. The victim's left hand is in a direct line with the mugger's groin. With this accomplished, the victim should extend all five fingers and reach back and grab the mugger's testicles—squeezing them as hard as he can. This counterattack will cause enough pain to make the mugger let go. As the yoke is released, the victim lunges forward and runs to safety.

No further fighting should take place. The mugger may recover in a few seconds and be able to resume the attack. He may have a concealed weapon or he may be aided by one or more companions. Once the victim is free, his only motive should be escape.

If you are caught in the yoke, when should you try to resist? The cue may come from the mugger. He may tell you that if you give up your belongings you won't be hurt. Or he may have a partner who will take your money while you are still in the mugger's grasp. If you are sure that the mugger is only after your property, it is not necessary to fight back.

But the yoke can also be used to drag you into a secluded place from which there is little chance of escape. This place may be your own home or apartment, a laundry room, an elevator, or a narrow alley way. You can try to pull away from the mugger, but the person applying the yoke has the advantage of leverage. Thus, as you try to lean forward, the mugger can use the yoke to pull your neck and shoulders back. The result of your efforts are tremendous pressure on your lower back and little, if any, movement in the right direction.

In this situation, I strongly advocate that you try to escape. Once the mugger has you where you can't be seen, he is free to commit any type of crime. His intentions may include more than robbery. You may be in danger of sexual abuse, further violence, or even murder. Where this is a possibility, I recommend that you try to get free.

A LIKELY STORY   Ken entered the elevator on the fifth floor and noticed a muscular young man standing in the corner. For some reason, Ken suspected that this man was a mugger. He secretly compared the man's strength with his own and wondered what would happen if the two of them were in a fight. While Ken daydreamed about this possibility, he was not really concerned. The man was no bigger than he was and did not appear to be armed. If the man *was* a criminal, he was probably waiting for a woman or an older tenant to board the elevator. Ken casually glanced over and tried to see if the young man was carrying a concealed weapon. At the same time, the young man noticed the wallet that was bulging prominently in **Ken's** back pocket.

On the third floor, the elevator stopped and another passenger got on. This man was the same age as the first. The two did not look at each other and not a word was spoken. With the entrance of this third person, Ken was secretly relieved. There was not much chance of his being attacked in the presence of a witness. He felt that he and this new passenger could certainly deal with the man he suspected—if that were necessary. Confident that he was safe, Ken stood in front of the elevator door and waited for it to open.

As the car landed on the main floor, Ken exited first and took one step toward the street. At that instant, he heard someone whisper "yoke him" and he knew that the two men were working together. It was too late to escape. The first mugger grabbed him around the throat (in the mugger's yoke) and tried to pull him back into the elevator. The second mugger held the door.

As Ken felt the arm squeeze tighter around his throat, he tried to bury his chin in his chest. Instinctively, his neck muscles strained against the mugger's arm. But this only made the pressure more severe.

After just a second, Ken thought he was going to suffocate. He twisted his neck slowly until he found a spot where he could breathe easier. His head was now almost at a right angle to its normal position.

Encouraged by the success of this move, Ken placed his right hand over the mugger's right elbow and started to push down. The mugger's arm budged just a fraction of an inch, but Ken could feel the difference. The pressure on his throat was almost completely relieved.

For the first time, however, he recognized a crisis of a different nature. In applying the yoke, the mugger had pulled so hard that Ken was almost lifted off his feet. Ever since then the mugger had been trying to pull him into the elevator and Ken had been unconsciously resisting.

Ken's feet had barely moved, but his head and shoulders had been yanked back so far that his body almost formed an arc. He could feel the muscles stretching in his lower back and he knew they could not endure much more. In a few seconds, he would have to relax and submit to the mugger. Ken was not ready to do this.

At this moment, he asked himself what was available and he thought of his left arm that was flailing uselessly in the air. His head was still turned to the right; but he knew if he was facing forward, his head and the mugger's would be in a line. He stretched out his thumb and thrust it back in the direction of the mugger's left eye. As he did this, he turned his head slightly so he could follow the blow.

When the thumb made contact, Ken could not tell if he had struck the eye, but he felt a slight loosening of the mugger's grip. This was a cue for action. Ken shifted his body to the right and reached down with his left hand and grabbed the mugger in the most sensitive area of the groin. This was enough to make the mugger let go. Ken pushed aside the arms that had been holding him and dashed quickly toward the door.

• • • Why didn't the mugger's companion help him? In this case, the victim was lucky. The mugger, himself, blocked his partner's view of what was happening. The partner never saw what the victim was doing with his left hand.

When the victim broke free, he had the advantage of surprise. He was able to get to the door before the mugger had recovered and before the partner realized that his friend had been hurt. If you were in this situation, would you have used force to get free? Would you have felt squeamish about grabbing the mugger's testicles?

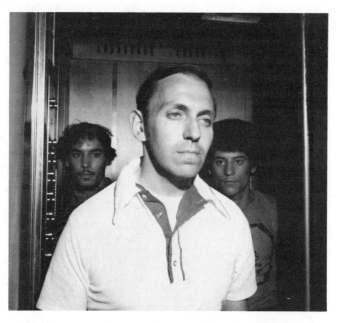

The elevator is a common site for indoor mugging.

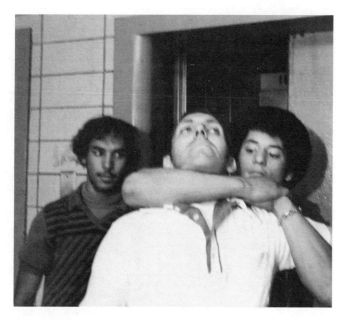

One mugger applies the yoke, while the other gets ready to hold the door.

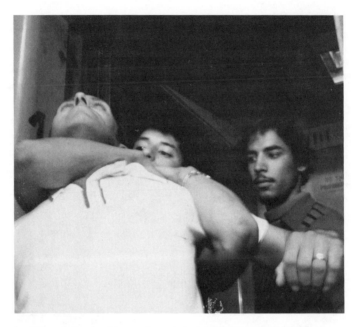

The victim is dragged back toward the open elevator.

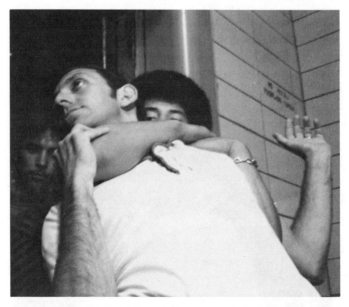

Fearing strangulation, the victim turns his head to the bend in the mugger's arm. In this position, there is less pressure on the windpipe.

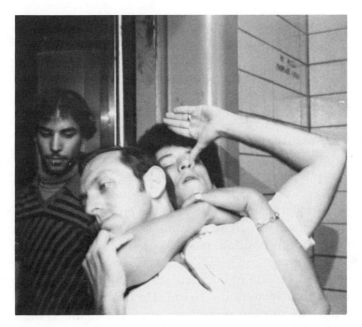

The victim pushes down on the arm around his neck. With the thumb of his other hand, he jabs the mugger in the eye.

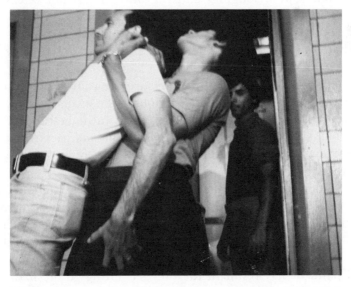

The next move is to shift the body to the right and to grab the mugger's testicles with the left hand.

Getting out of the Headlock

The headlock is a useful device for the mugger who operates alone. Only one arm is needed to apply this grip. The mugger's other arm is free to remove the victim's belongings or to strike the victim if he or she offers resistance.

The headlock has other advantages for the criminal. For example, it is a good means of intimidating a victim. If you were caught in this hold, your head would be squeezed between the bend in the mugger's arm and his chest. As the mugger tightened his grip, you would experience some discomfort and find it impossible to squirm free. In this position, most people feel trapped and are quite willing to cooperate.

Another advantage of the headlock is that it gives the mugger an opportunity to maneuver the victim. He can pull the victim to the front or the back or exert pressure to lower the victim to the ground.

The guidelines for fighting back are the same as for most other holds. If the mugger is only after your property, it is probably best to submit and to give the mugger what he wants. However, if you have surrendered your belongings and the mugger has not released his grip, it is probably a good idea to consider resistance.

If you decide to resist, what will you have available? You will immediately recognize that your hands and arms are free. The problem is how to use them effectively.

If you are bothered by the pressure on your head, your first reaction may be to use your hands to loosen the mugger's grip. As we have seen with other holds, this is usually a futile gesture. It is not likely that you can grab the mugger's arm and remove it from around your head. A better approach would be to use your hands to attack the mugger in other areas.

One device that is often successful is the "famous Griffith pinch." (Many a rambunctious recruit from the police academy can attest to the effectiveness of this measure.) To apply the pinch, you should slide your hand behind the mugger's legs and grab the skin on the inside of his left or right thigh. This will cause a sharp, unexpected pain. It may result in the mugger letting go or, at the least, relaxing his grip.

You can position your hand for the pinch without the mugger

detecting this movement. For one thing, you are attacking the mugger from behind. Another factor in your favor is that the mugger will not be watching your hands. He will probably be concentrating on the headlock or, if he is going to move you, he will be looking in the direction where he wants to go. The fact that the pinch comes as a surprise makes it even more effective.

If this technique does not allow you to break the hold, your next move should be toward the mugger's groin. Step forward with the foot that is further away from your assailant. If he is holding you in his right arm, step forward with your right foot and reach for his testicles with your right hand. Squeeze hard and get ready to break free.

This is what should happen. As the grip around your head was being tightened, the mugger was bending forward and was forcing your head closer to his body. The pain inflicted by the pinch or the hold on his testicles should cause the mugger to straighten up. When he does, the separation between his arm and body will be greater and there will be more room for your head. If at this point, you cannot slide out of the hold, you can use your right hand to further loosen the grip. Slip your hand between your head and the mugger's forearm and push the mugger's arm away. The moment you can move your head, either duck down under the mugger's grip or pull back and away. Once you are free, start to run.

The important things to remember are:

1. Use your hands, but don't try to grab the mugger's arm and pull it off your head.
2. Reach behind the mugger's leg and pinch him on the inside of the thigh. This is a sensitive spot that will be black and blue for several days.
3. Step forward with your outside leg (not the leg that is next to the mugger) and grab the mugger's testicles with your outside hand.
4. Step 2 or Step 3—or a combination of both—should cause the mugger to straighten up and loosen his grip. If you are still unable to squirm free, get your hand inside the mugger's grip and push his arm away from his body.
5. As you perform Step 4, move your head down or back until it is completely removed from the mugger's hold.

The sixth step you should know by heart. As soon as you are free, run as fast as you can and yell for help. Don't stand around to recover your belongings.

A LIKELY STORY The Suburban Company (the name is fictitious) has a large staff of weekday workers. But on Saturdays the only people who are expected in the office are part-time employees who do typing and filing. Since the building is almost empty, Suburban locks all their entrances except one. This door is attended by a watchman or by a member of the maintenance staff. As people enter through this door, they are required to sign a log.

These security measures appear to be adequate, but unfortunately the doors to Suburban are easy to unlock. This was proven on a Saturday afternoon in July when a mugger strolled through the parking lot and approached a pair of glass doors that were marked "Employees." The doors had been locked during the previous evening, but the mugger slipped a knife in between them and used this knife to depress the latch. He entered quietly and stationed himself in a corner. There he remained for a few minutes until he saw a lone employee who was walking outside. Her name was Noreen and she had been with the company for just a few weeks.

She had left work through the only attended door and was walking along side the building to get to her car. As she passed the employee's entrance, the glass door opened behind her and she was grabbed by the mugger. Before she could get away, he had wrapped his right arm around her head and was squeezing it tightly. With his other hand, he reached over and slipped her pocketbook off her shoulder. He held this by the strap as he continued to tighten his grip.

From Noreen's point of view, the loss of the pocketbook was minor. What she did care about was getting free. The mugger had lowered her head until it was no higher than the rest of her body. This caused her back to be bent at a right angle and the only way she could keep it from aching was by trying to relax. She made an effort to do this, but she couldn't keep the muscles in her back from tightening up.

The discomfort in her back, however, was secondary compared to the pain inflicted by the headlock. Her right ear felt like it was crushed. Her cheekbones grew sore from the closeness of the mugger's grip. But even this sensation could not compare to the queasiness she felt because she was unable to move her head. The thought kept coming back to her, "If he wants to hit me in the face, I can't get out of the way."

Noreen didn't think about the mugger's intentions—why he was still holding her or what he planned to do next. Her only concern was getting out of the headlock. In desperation, she decided to try something she had read about in a magazine. She looked down at the mugger's legs and reached behind them with her left hand. Although she couldn't follow the movement of this hand with her eyes, she was able to place it on the back of the mugger's left thigh and to dig the sharp nails of the thumb and forefinger into the soft flesh in the back of his leg.

The mugger's reaction to this pinch was to grunt loudly and to straighten up. As he did, he loosened the grip around Noreen's head. She continued to attack by stepping forward with her right leg and reaching for his groin with her right hand. The mugger was too slow to protect himself. He was holding Noreen with one arm and hanging onto her bag with the other. Thus, he could not use his hands to stop her from grabbing his testicles. She squeezed hard and the mugger pulled back in pain. As he did, the arm that was bent around her head straightened slightly. Noreen was able to get her right hand inside his grip and to push his forearm away from his body. This opened the headlock and allowed her to duck under his arm. She left the mugger holding her pocketbook and ran through the lot until she reached an open gas station. There she made a phone call and waited for the police.

• • • Let us briefly review the action of the story. Our first observation is that the Suburban Company did not protect their weekend employees as well as they thought. A lock guard could have prevented the mugger from opening the doors with a knife. If he had been able to enter, his presence could have been detected if the burglar alarm on the door had been hooked up. There is not much that Noreen could have done to avoid being mugged—except that she would have been safer if she had left the building with another employee.

Why the mugger continued to apply the headlock after he had Noreen's pocketbook is not clear. But the possibilities are frightening. He may have planned to hurt her so she could not go back into the building and summon help. Or he may have wanted to wrestle her to the ground and molest her sexually. Or his motive may have even been abduction. Whatever his reasons, Noreen appeared to make the right decision in fighting back.

I'm sure you noticed that when Noreen got free she didn't try to get back her pocketbook. She also didn't risk getting into her car or trying to get back inside the building. In either situation, she may have been caught as she was trying to get in the door.

How would you compare the security of the Suburban Company to the protection that is provided by your own employer or landlord? How does it compare to the safety of your own home? Could a burglar open your door with just a small knife? If so, you may want to invest in a lock guard, a chain, or even an alarm. These devices may not keep out every burglar, but they will deter most criminals from breaking in.

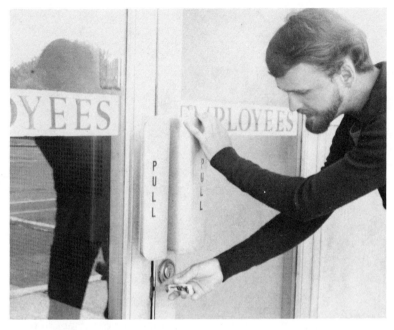

A locked door does not deter the experienced criminal.

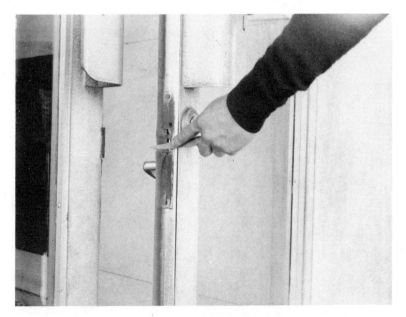

He depresses the latch with a knife and waits inside for an unsuspecting victim.

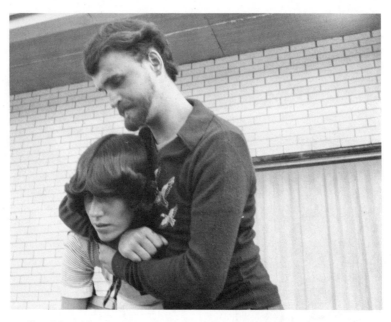

Catching his victim by surprise, the mugger grabs her in a headlock. With his other hand, he slips her pocketbook off her arm.

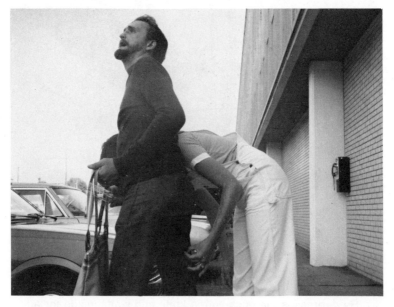

The mugger is startled by a pinch on the back of his thigh.

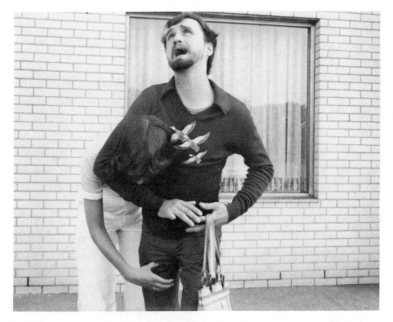

The victim steps forward with her right foot and reaches for the groin with her right hand.

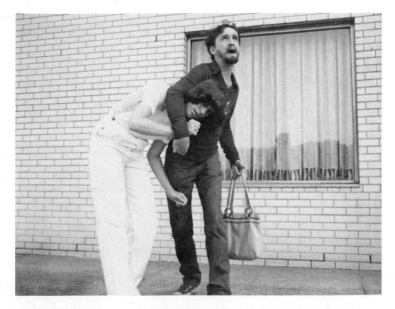

In considerable pain, the mugger loosens his grip. This is the victim's opportunity to open the headlock and slip away.

Breaking out of the Bear Hug

The bear hug is a simple hold in which the attacker wraps his arms around the victim's arms and torso and squeezes tightly. This grip can be applied from the front or rear.

In the heyday of TV wrestling, a giant wrestler would get his opponent in this hold, lift him off the ground, and squeeze until the opponent went limp. Then the wrestler would drop the unconscious opponent to the mat, pounce on top of him for three sounds, and win the match.

If you were caught in a bear hug on the street, you would not have to worry about being squeezed until you were unconscious. Your main concern would be abduction. The attacker is probably using this grip to remove you to a place where you can't be seen. If this is the situation, he is probably after you rather than your property. His motivation may be kidnapping, physical abuse, or rape.

The use of the bear hug would most likely warrant resistance. You have been trained to ask yourself "What is available?" In this case, what you do not have available are your arms. They are pinned to your side and while you can move your hands up and down, you cannot move your arms away from your body. This is difficult, because when you think of self-defense your arms are what you usually think of first.

Let us examine the escape from the bear hug that is applied from the front. The attacker is facing you and his arms are squeezed around your body. As he tightens his grip, he is leaning against you and pushing you back. What would be your reaction?

The normal response is to fight force with force. The bear hug is pressing in on your arms and chest. The usual tendency is to try to expand your chest and push your arms back and out in an attempt to break the hold. You may have seen this work on TV wrestling, but for you to do this successfully, you would have to be considerably stronger than your opponent. It is probably better to resist the temptation to use your arms and to concentrate on what you do have available.

Two things that are available to you are your hands and feet. You do not have complete use of your hands, but you can raise them slightly. This is all you will need to effectively disable your attacker.

Let your hands remain close together in front of your body. Curl your fingers, as if you were making a fist, but do not bend your thumbs. These should be pointed up and toward your attacker. When you are ready to fight back, jab both thumbs into your attacker's testicles. At the same time, lift one foot a few inches off the ground and slam your heel into your assailant's instep. The combination of these blows should be enough to loosen the grip. As you feel the bear hug relaxed, push free—to the right or left—and run.

In most situations, it would be difficult to land a blow to the groin. Men may be accidentally injured in this area, but deliberate strikes to the groin are seldom successful. This is because men will instinctively protect themselves from any punch or kick that comes near this sensitive part of the body. When you are in the bear hug, however, your hands are concealed from your attacker. Thus, he cannot see the blow and he will not have a chance to cover up.

While this may be the best way to break the bear hug, it is not the only means of escape. In 1975, a woman in the Sheepshead Nostrand development in Brooklyn was caught in this hold. She managed to get free and then summoned the police. When they arrived, she could not give them a detailed description of her attacker. She had forgotten his age, size, attire, and facial features. The only thing she could remember to tell them was "Look for a black man with a bite on his cheek." The woman had remembered that her teeth were available and had used them to get free. While it is unpleasant to think about biting another human being, in an emergency this is an acceptable means of defense.

You will have to use different techniques if you are caught in a bear hug that is applied from the rear. As with the front bear hug, your arms may be immobilized but your hands and feet will be free. The question is "How will you use them?"

One thing you can do is to swing your foot back so that your heel strikes the attacker's shin. If you are accurate, this can be a painful experience for the person who is kicked. However, if you are being pulled back, there is a fair chance that you will not make contact or that you will kick your attacker on the side of the leg. For this reason, I suggest that you first try to use your hands.

Having answered the question "What do I have available?" you might now ask yourself, "Where can my attacker be hurt?"

It may be that you cannot reach his groin or eyes. This will be the case if your arms are locked in the bear hug. What you will be able to reach, however, are the attacker's fingers and arms. These can provide you with a quick way out of the hold.

One means of escape is to grab the small finger of the hand that is on top and pull it back and *away* from your body. (If the mugger's right hand is on top, grab his right pinky in your right hand. Use both hands if necessary.) As the finger is pulled back, the rest of the arm should follow. This would open up the bear hug and allow you to get free. If the attacker tried to keep his arm in place, the finger would be pulled back to the point of breaking. The intensity of the pain would cause him to relax his grip, and you would have a chance to step out and get away.

Another technique that is easy to apply is the pinch. Your attacker's arms are right in front of you. With your thumb and forefinger about $\frac{1}{4}$ inch apart, grab the skin on either arm and squeeze hard. Preferably, you should choose a spot near the bend of the arm, where there is more flesh and the skin is loose.

The pinch will not disable a person, but it will cause a sudden pain that is much like a bee sting. Since the attacker is not expecting this, he will be both hurt and startled. The usual reaction is to jump back and move the arm that has been pinched. When this happens, you have the opportunity to break the hold.

The pinch is a good example of getting the maximum effect out of the minimum effort. Many people will try to use their nails to scratch their attacker. While scratching can be painful, it does not have the immediate impact of a simple pinch.

JUDY'S STORY It was a Saturday afternoon and Judy was on her way to visit a friend. Since she was a few minutes early, she decided to cut through the park. She was walking slowly across a lawn, when she was greeted by a friendly looking stranger. "Excuse me, miss," he asked, "Do you have the time? My watch seems to have stopped."

"Sure," Judy obliged. She was not expecting any danger as she glanced down at her wrist. But the minute she looked away from the stranger, she felt his arms knot around her waist. Worse than this, her own arms were pinned at her side. For a moment, she felt defenseless.

Although it was daytime, the park was in a business area and since this was a weekend there was no one else around. Shouting would not do any good. No one would hear and it might cause the attacker to become violent.

The man was considerably taller than Judy. He leaned forward and buried his right shoulder in her chest and was about to push her back. Another girl might have been helpless, but Judy had two older brothers who had prepared her for just this type of situation.

Knowing what to do, she remained confident. Her arms were still locked at her side, but she tested her hands and saw that she could move them up or down a few inches. When she realized this, she clenched her fists and kept them in front of her body. As the attacker got ready to push her, Judy pointed her thumbs directly at his groin. The attacker did not notice. He was looking over her shoulder to the place where he was going to move.

Judy knew what she was going to do; it was just a matter of when. Suddenly, a voice inside her whispered "now," and as if she was responding to that command, Judy straightened up and jabbed both thumbs into the attacker's groin. The man doubled over and stretched out his arms. Before he had felt the full impact of the blow, Judy struck again. This time she lifted her heel and plunged it straight down on the mugger's instep.

Her next move was to turn to the right and to brush aside the man's arms. By now his arms were no longer wrapped around her; they were just leaning on her body. The moment she was free from the man's touch, she started to run, and she didn't stop until she was on the other side of the park—a few hundred yards away. When she got to the edge of the park, she looked around for the first time. The man had not followed her. He was walking away in the other direction.

Judy was out of breath, but she still managed to smile. "My brothers would be proud of me" she thought. Then she continued on to her friend's house and got ready to tell the whole story.

• • • If Judy were your sister or daughter, would you have taught her how to defend herself? If you were Judy, would you have been interested in learning self-defense or would you have considered these tactics unfeminine?

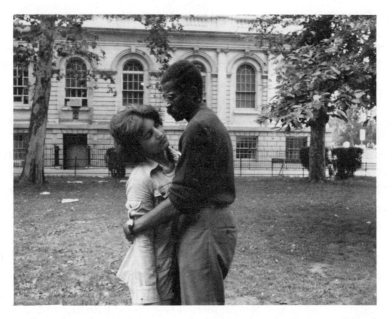

The victim's upper arms are immobilized but both of her hands are free.

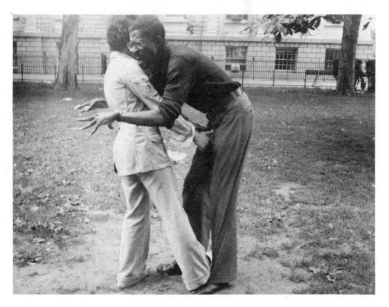

She points her thumbs toward the mugger's groin and jabs them into his testicles. At the same time, she slams into his instep with the heel of her shoe.

LADONNA'S STORY   As Ladonna walked through the subway turnstile, she saw a man standing next to the steps that led outside. She was mildly suspicious, but she scolded herself for being afraid. The man looked in her direction and Ladonna smiled back politely. A moment later, she was starting to climb the steps.

As she reached the fourth step, the man bounded onto the stair behind her and grabbed her tightly around the waist. The firmness of his grip made Ladonna gasp for air. She heard him say something in a foreign language and then he tried to drag her back inside the station. Ladonna wished that she had not been traveling alone.

Although the man's grip was only around her waist, she did not realize that her arms were free. She was waving them wildly in the air to maintain her balance, but she was only thinking about her feet and their struggle to hold the ground. As the man pulled back, Ladonna's right hand latched onto the bannister. She held on tight to keep herself from being dragged back down the stairs.

Feeling resistance for the first time, the man tugged harder to get Ladonna away from the bannister. As he did, Ladonna's left hand brushed against his face. This made her realize that her hands were available and that she could use them to protect herself.

She looked down and saw her attacker's arms around her waist. They were unprotected. Ladonna didn't know it, but the attacker was looking the other way. He was trying to pull her down and he was watching the steps between himself and the landing.

There were tricks Ladonna had learned as a little girl when she had wrestled with her older brothers. They were bigger and stronger than she was, but when they got too rough she had ways of getting free. One thing that always worked was a good hard pinch.

With this in mind, she moved her right hand off the bannister and grabbed the man's flesh right near the crook of the elbow. She pinched hard and the man yelped in surprise. He loosened his grip, but he didn't let go.

There were other tricks that Ladonna remembered. She reached over with the same hand and grabbed the man's right pinky. She pulled it back as far as she could, and as she did she drew his hand away from her body. The man was momentarily stunned by the pain in his arm and finger. Meanwhile, Ladonna slithered through his grip and ran up the steps. As she reached the top, she started to yell "police." The man turned around and ran back into the station.

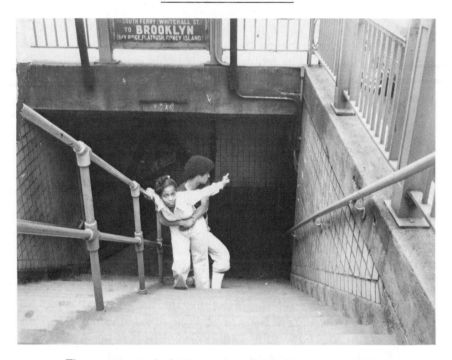

The mugger grabs Ladonna from behind and starts to drag her down the steps.

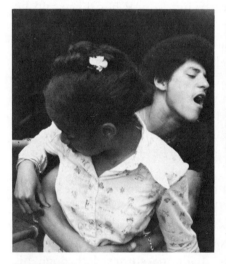

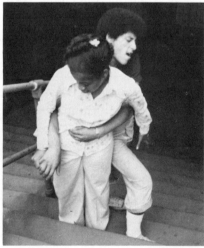

Realizing that her hands are available, Ladonna pinches the mugger in a sensitive spot.

She grabs the mugger's small finger and pulls back as hard as she can. By doing this, she breaks the hold.

Breaking the Stranglehold

In this section, we will talk about two grips: one where the attacker's arms are straight and one where his elbows are bent. In both cases, the attacker is facing the victim and his hands are around the victim's throat. Quite often the person being choked is shoved back against a wall. When this happens, the attacker leans forward and puts all his weight on his arms. The pressure against the victim's throat is greatly increased. The force of the stranglehold keeps the victim pinned against the wall.

The attacker's frame of mind may be different when he applies the stranglehold than when he has the victim in another grip. The purpose of this hold may originally be to scare a victim or to throttle a person into submission. But as the attacker tightens his grip, his motivation may change. He may feel a strange sense of power in knowing that he can squeeze the life out of a victim. Or, if he is choking a woman, he may try to strangle her to prove that he is physically superior. In some ways, the motives of the strangler and the rapist may be the same.

The use of the stranglehold is seldom premeditated. It may be applied by a frustrated mugger or rapist, or may even be used as the result of a family argument. More often than not, women are the victims of this hold.

Suppose you were caught in this hold. When you first felt the strangler's fingers pressing into your throat, what would you do? The most usual reaction would be to grab your attacker's hands and to try to pull them off your throat. This move sometimes excites the strangler just as begging may urge the predatory mugger to become more violent. At the same time, the attempt to pull off the mugger's hands is usually futile. It requires too much strength.

Rather than grab the strangler's hands or wrists, you should concentrate on the elbows. If your attacker's arms are straight, bring your hands up outside his elbows and hit both of them at the same time with your palms. As you do this, straighten your arms and push back. This is what you accomplish:

By driving the strangler's elbows in, you are forcing his hands out and causing him to release the grip. Remember that the strangler uses his arms to lean his weight against you. Once you get his hands off your neck, he is off balance. As you push back on his elbows, it is easy to push him away.

There are two steps to this technique. The first is to hit the attacker's elbows with your palms and to force them in. The second is to straighten your arms and push back. One move follows immediately after the other. For both moves, the point of contact is the strangler's elbows.

Please note that the elbows should be hit rather than pushed. It will take a fair amount of force to break the hold. I am often asked if there is any way that the strangler can prevent you from hitting his elbows. I can't think of any, since both of his hands are gripping your neck. The only way for him to avoid the blow is to release the grip.

When you push the mugger back, you will be leaning forward. Start to run in the direction in which you are leaning. In other words, you should try to run around the strangler instead of turning around and running in the opposite direction. You would lose time in turning and would be more likely to be caught.

A different technique is needed if the strangler's elbows are bent. In this position, the strangler's body is much closer to you and his arms are spread wide apart. Once again he is leaning forward so the force of his weight is pressing against you.

As before, your keys to freedom are the strangler's elbows. Cup your hands so that you form a 'U' with your thumb and forefinger. Then raise both hands at the same time. As you hit the strangler's elbows, push them up and away. A moderate amount of force will release the grip and send the strangler flying back. As you get free, do not stop to admire your handiwork. Run past the strangler and yell for help.

Please note the difference between the two techniques. In the first situation, the strangler's elbows are facing out and you are pushing them in. In the second case, the strangler's elbows are pointing down and you are forcing them up. The second part of both techniques is the same. In both instances, your hands are on the strangler's elbows and you are pushing him away.

TWO STORIES WITH THE SAME ENDING Susan was sitting alone in the park when she noticed a man watching her. The man's gaze made her uncomfortable; she tried to look away, but she could still tell that his eyes were fixed on her. Trying to look natural, she glanced at her watch and rose slowly. She continued to move at a relaxed pace toward the street. She didn't want the man to think that she was running away.

Unknown to Susan, there were two exits from the park. When she got half way to the street, the man leaped up and light-footed it to the other exit. He was able to get out of the park and turn the corner so that he met Susan face-to-face on the street.

"How about it?" the man grinned.

Susan looked away. "Please, leave me alone," she said.

"C'mon," the man persisted.

"No," she answered as she tried to brush him aside.

The man would not be put off that easily. He grabbed her by the neck and shoved her against the wall of a wooden newspaper stand. As Susan tried to get free, he tightened his grip so she was pinned against the wall.

The man was not planning to attack, but the frightened look in Susan's eyes impressed him. He could feel his fingers squeezing into her neck and he knew it was hard for her to breathe. She was completely under his control.

Susan, in the meantime, was desperate to get free. She tugged at the strangler's wrists, but they wouldn't budge. She knew this type of escape would be impossible, but she was encouraged by the fact that her hands were free. The strangler's arms were longer than hers and she could not conveniently reach his body to strike him in the eyes or groin. What she did instead was raise her hands with her fingers pointing upward. When her hands were even with the strangler's elbows, she clapped them together. As the man's elbows moved in, his hands spread apart. This left the strangler shaky since he had been leaning forward. Susan was still holding his elbows and she had an easy time as she pushed him back and away.

When Susan got free, about 6 feet separated her from the strangler. She whispered to herself "Thank God" and then lunged forward and ran past her attacker. The man was shocked by his own actions and by Susan's sudden escape. By the time he turned to chase after her, Susan had enough of a head start to get safely away.

Let us alter that story just slightly. Suppose that when Susan was forced against the wall, the strangler moved himself closer so he was just a few inches away from her. In this position, the strangler's elbows were bent and they were separated by at least the width of his shoulders.

Susan looked away for fear of looking her attacker in the eye. But peripherally she got a view of the strangler's arms and could see the spot where each was bent. Instead of moving her hands to the outside—as she did in the first story—she readied them beneath his elbows. The strangler did not see this move, as he was staring at her face. He was caught completely by surprise when he was struck on the elbows and shoved back. Susan had hit his elbows and had grabbed them at the same time. As she pushed up and away, the man's hands flew up and he stumbled backwards. He was still off balance as Susan darted around him and continued running.

• • • What is your opinion? Could Susan have kept this man from using force? Suppose she had said she was waiting for her husband— do you think that would have made a difference?

Some people ask me if by resisting the strangler they are endangering their own lives. My reply is "Sure, the strangler may be angry and may try to kill you. But what was he trying to do in the first place?"

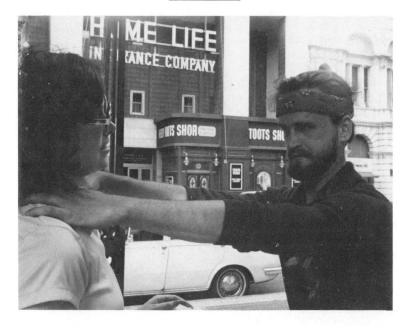

Susan is pinned against the solid wall of a newspaper stand. The strangler is leaning forward and his arms are straight.

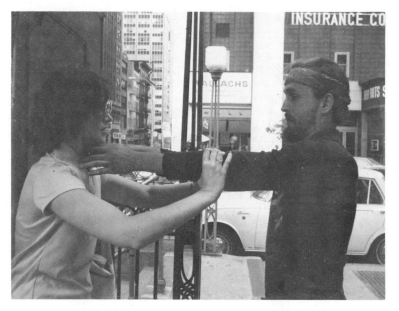

When Susan pushes in on the strangler's elbows, his hands spread apart.

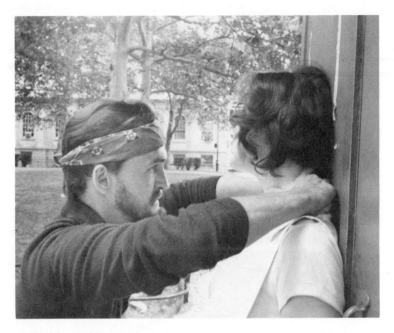

In this scene, the strangler has moved closer to Susan and his arms are bent.

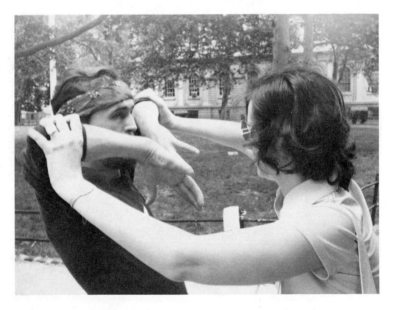

Susan lifts his arms from the elbows and pushes the strangler back and away.

Defending Yourself Against the Female Criminal

Many of the muggers I have interviewed consider the female criminal to be even more dangerous than the male. In their opinion, she is more likely to injure a victim without provocation. What special techniques are needed to deal with this type of mugger?

As always, the best protection is being alert. Too often we let down our guard in the presence of females because we don't expect them to attack. When we are not careful, we are an easy prey for the female mugger.

Being robbed by a woman may be embarrassing for a male victim. But he should respond to this mugger in the same way he would respond to her male counterpart. There is no disgrace in not offering resistance.

When force is necessary, the male victim may find it difficult to strike a woman. But this is socially acceptable when the alternative is to suffer a serious injury. When force must be used, it is important to remember that a woman is particularly sensitive in the area of her stomach and her breasts. The following story gives one example of how a victim can defend himself against a female attacker.

A LIKELY STORY   Vinnie did not take unnecessary chances. When he was aware of danger, he avoided it. This particular afternoon, he had walked into a garden behind a large office building. The garden was empty except for two girls who were coming down a nearby path. Vinnie saw the girls, but did not think of them as a threat to his safety. As he walked past them, one of the girls grabbed him from behind. She held his head in both hands and at the same time covered his mouth. The other girl took hold of his collar and aimed a large stick at the exposed area of his head. Without asking for his money, his watch, or any valuables, the girl raised the stick and prepared to strike.

Vinnie had the advantage of size, but the girls outnumbered him and one of them was armed. His best course of action was to try to escape. To do this, he shifted his body to the right, so that it was no longer shielding the girl behind him. As he moved away, he jabbed his left elbow to the rear. He watched it from the corner of his eye and saw it strike the girl in the pit of the stomach. She doubled over and loosened the grip around his head. Before she could regain her hold, Vinnie had straightened up and had thrust his elbow back into her breasts. While he did this with his left arm, he used the two front fingers of his right hand to poke the eyes of the girl in front of him. He succeeded in disabling both women—at least temporarily—but he did not stay to continue the battle. Without embarrassment, he ran through the garden and yelled for help.

• • • Muggers often attack in pairs so that one person can hold the victim while the other can search for money or beat the victim into submission. If you are sandwiched between two attackers, you must first concentrate on the one who is holding you. After you have broken free, you can deal with his (or her) companion.

In preparing to strike the girl behind him, Vinnie kept his feet in place but shifted his torso to the right. Had he stepped to the right, the girl would have moved with him and would have remained directly behind his body. In this position, she would not have been hit in the stomach or breasts.

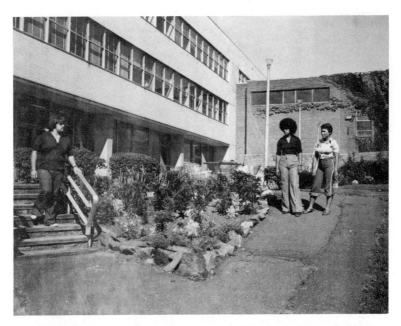

In the presence of two young women, Vinnie does not sense that he is in danger.

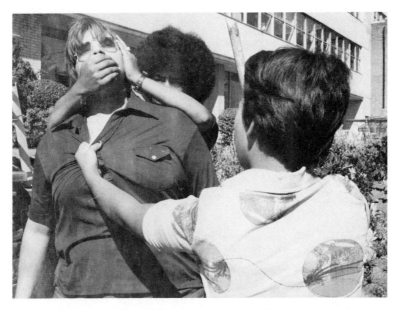

One mugger grabs him from behind, while the other prepares to hit him with a stick.

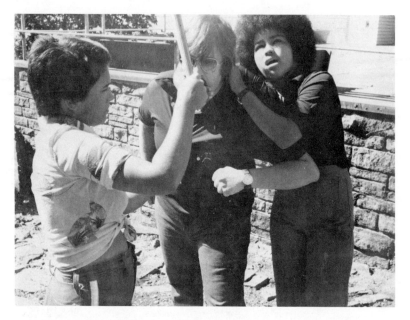

Vinnie shifts his body to the right so he can hit the girl who is holding him. He thrusts his elbow into her stomach.

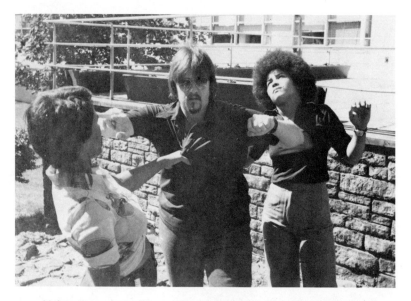

Using the same elbow, Vinnie strikes the girl behind him in the breasts. With his right hand, he pokes the other girl in the eyes.

Using a Cane or Umbrella for Protection

Let us think back to the key to safety—the question "What do I have available?" Sometimes the answer to that question is very obvious. You may be carrying an umbrella or using a cane for support. Both of these implements can be used as weapons. Before I explain their use, however, let me offer you one note of caution.

Any weapon in your possession can be taken away from you and used against you. Therefore, it is important that before you defend yourself with your cane or umbrella, you make sure that their use is necessary. I would not depend on them to protect my property. I would only use them to protect myself from serious injury.

Because you don't want to lose possession of your cane or umbrella, it is important that you employ them carefully and effectively. There are two different methods of using them. The method you choose should depend on whether or not the mugger is armed.

If the mugger is not carrying a knife, a club, or a gun, you will want to use your own weapon (your cane or umbrella) like a bayonet. For the purpose of instruction, let us assume that you are walking with a cane. To use it against an assailant, you should position your body so you are not facing him directly. If you are holding the cane in your right hand, turn so that your left hip is pointed a few degrees to the left of the attacker. Lift the cane so it is parallel to the ground or pointed up slightly. The tip of your cane should be aimed at the person you are going to hit.

Remember that you are holding the handle in your right hand; your left hand should grab the stem of the cane near the tip. It is the job of this hand to direct the cane.

When you are ready to strike the attacker, jab the tip of the cane toward his eyes, throat, stomach, or groin. Your right hand should be thrusting the cane forward and your left hand should be guiding it to the area that you are going to hit. As soon as you make contact, pull back and strike again. While you are jabbing the mugger, you should be calling for help. Your screaming may bring you assistance and it will also help you to summon up extra strength.

Once you feel that the mugger is disabled or off balance, try to get away. Do not become overconfident and continue the attack. Even though you have your cane for protection, you are still in danger. If you have an opportunity to escape, your should certainly do so.

These techniques can be used against more than one attacker at a time. For example, in 1976, Boston Riley, an 82-year-old resident of the Bronx, was trapped in a laundry room by three assailants. Despite his age, he was able to use his cane to keep his attackers at bay. Eventually he managed to get out of the laundry room without being hurt.

When you are defending yourself against more than one person, it is important that you don't let any of your attackers get behind you. If they do, they will be able to grab you without being struck by your cane. Sometimes it may be necessary to retreat against a door or a wall so there is no possibility of being attacked from behind.

You have probably wondered if you wouldn't be more successful if you were swinging your cane like a baseball bat. This is not a good idea for a few reasons.

1. When you swing a cane, you are less likely to hit the mugger in a sensitive area. While you might aim your swing at the mugger's head, there is more of a chance that you will hit him in the arm or shoulder and do little damage. With this type of attack, the mugger is better able to avoid your blows.
2. While you may have confidence in your ability to hurt the mugger in this way, most people who swing a cane cannot get much force behind their swing.
3. When you are holding the cane near the handle, the person you are striking has a chance to grab it by the stem. If he succeeds in doing this, he may be able to pull it away from you.

For these reasons, the bayonet approach is preferred. However, there are circumstances where the bayonet approach should not be used.

For the mugger who is holding a knife, a different technique is needed. If you were to thrust at him, you would bring yourself closer to the knife and would increase your chance of being stabbed. What you want to accomplish in this situation is to get the knife out of the mugger's hand. Once again you can use your cane. But this time instead of jabbing at the mugger's body, you will be striking down at the hand that is holding the weapon. One blow may not be enough. You will have to continue hitting his hand until he lets go of the knife.

When protecting yourself against the armed mugger, you should hold the cane in your stronger hand or, if possible, in both hands. You may be able to control the cane better if you hold it a few inches above the handle—by doing this, you will be "choking up" on it just like a batter "chokes up" on a baseball bat. But don't shorten the cane by too much. Its length gives you an advantage. It allows you to strike the mugger while you are still a safe distance from his knife.

Separating the mugger from his knife is a big step toward safety. The mugger is still dangerous when he is not armed. But most criminals who carry a weapon rely on that weapon for confidence and protection. If it is taken away from them, they tend to lose their self-assurance.

Thus, if the mugger's knife is on the ground and you are yelling for help, the mugger may decide to turn and run. If he does, do not try to go after him. Remember the rule we established at the beginning of this chapter: The purpose of using force is to escape without being hurt.

A LIKELY STORY   Tina was a retired school teacher who could walk quite well with the help of a cane. One Tuesday she attended a senior citizens meeting at the community center. After the meeting was over, she stopped into their phone booth and called her doctor for an appointment. When she left the booth, she looked in only one direction and did not notice a man who was loitering in the halls. The man crept up behind her and whisked her pocketbook off her arm. As this happened, Tina instinctively turned toward the man and stared directly at him. Before she realized what she was doing, she had scowled at him and, in a scolding voice, she had yelled out "thief." Tina immediately knew that this was a mistake.

The man, angered by her response, was preparing to strike her with her own bag. He had raised it over his head and was aiming it down at her face. Tina knew that she would have to react quickly. She asked herself what she had available and she immediately thought of the cane she was holding in her right hand.

As the man stared down at her, Tina quickly shifted her position so that her left hip was pointing slightly to the left of the man. She raised her cane until it was almost at shoulder level. Then, she grabbed its stem in her left hand, and pointed its tip directly at the man's eyes. Before he could protect himself, Tina had poked the cane directly in the area where she was aiming. The man's head shot back with pain as he stumbled backwards. Tina did not wait to hit him again and did not try to recover her pocketbook. She hobbled down the hall and started yelling for help.

• • • Tina let down her guard when she came out of the phone booth. Had she looked both ways she might have noticed the purse snatcher.

When her bag was taken, she didn't try to hold onto it. But she couldn't resist the opportunity to scold the man who was robbing her. Many older people will do this. They will reprimand a criminal and make him even more hostile.

If you were carrying an umbrella, would you try to use it for protection? What other potential weapons might you have with you—a lit cigar, a pocketbook, a brief case? These are things that you might consider when you ask yourself "What do I have available?"

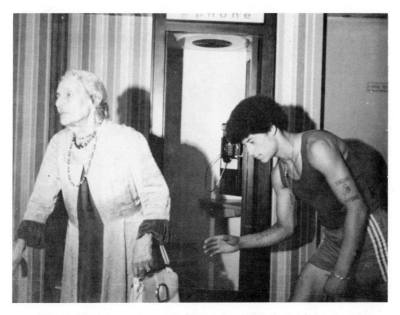

When Tina leaves the phone booth, she only looks in one direction. A would-be purse snatcher approaches from behind.

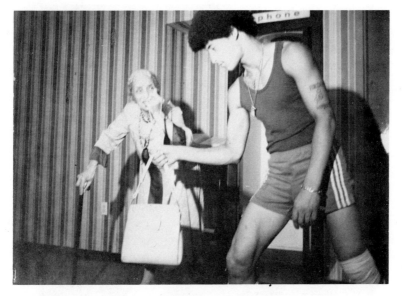

The purse snatcher succeeds in getting her bag, but Tina spots him in the act and calls him a thief.

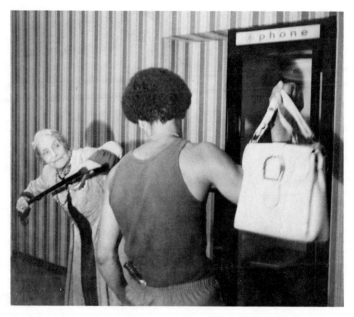

Angered by her remark, the man prepares to hit the victim with her own pocketbook. Tina holds her cane like a bayonet and aims it at the young man's eyes.

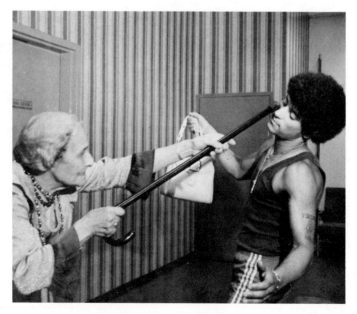

Tina jabs the tip of the cane into the man's right eye.

RESISTING THE MUGGER WHO IS ARMED

Early in this chapter, I suggested that the purpose of using force is to escape from a mugger before you are harmed. When you fight back against a mugger with a weapon, you must do more than just get away. It is necessary to get the weapon out of his hands.

The obvious reason for doing this is to prevent the mugger from using the weapon against you the moment you are free. A more subtle reason for separating the mugger from his knife or gun is that this object may be the root of his confidence. Once the weapon is not available, he may be less bold and less inclined to pursue the crime.

If you are threatened by an armed criminal, your predicament is extremely dangerous but it is not hopeless. The techniques you are going to learn have actually worked. However, they require careful practice and they should only be used as a last resort.

Survival with a Knife at Your Throat

When muggers are armed, the weapon that they choose most often is the knife. They may point this anywhere at the victim's body, but in most instances they want to be behind the victim and close enough to place the knife against the victim's throat. In this situation, the victim cannot afford to make a mistake—one wrong move and the mugger may use his weapon.

In earlier chapters, I stressed the importance of remaining calm. This may be your best defense when you are being robbed at knife-point. Suppose you are grabbed from behind by a mugger who places a knife along side your neck. Your first reaction may be to scream or to try to break free. But both of these responses are extremely dangerous. The last thing you want to do is to panic the mugger.

What I recommend in this situation is that you remain perfectly still and talk in a quiet voice. You might say to the mugger, "Please take my wallet, but leave my papers." This accomplishes a few things: (1) The mugger has had to strain to hear what you are saying. Thus, he is temporarily distracted. At least for the moment, he is not thinking about using the knife. (2) Another advantage to this approach is that you are telling the mugger that he can have your money. There is no need for him to use force. (3) By asking the mugger to leave your identification, you are demonstrating that you are still thinking clearly. Hopefully, your calm and rational approach will elicit the same type of response from the mugger.

Remember in Chapter 2 I mentioned that some muggers may actually be more scared than their victims. If this type of mugger is carrying a knife, you don't want to startle him with any quick moves or loud noises.

While it is certainly hoped that you will not have to use force, it is still necessary to be prepared. While you are talking to the mugger, keep one hand in the vicinity of his groin. The mugger will be watching your lips as you talk and he will also have an eye on his weapon. It is very unlikely that he will notice the position of your hand. Even if he does, he will not recognize it as a threat.

Do not try to grab the mugger unless you are positive that he is going to use his knife. If you are left with no alternative, squeeze his testicles hard and move quickly out of his grasp.

If you are approached from behind by a female mugger wielding a knife, the same type of response is wanted—except now you should keep one arm bent so that your elbow is pointing at the midsection of the mugger. Women are generally sensitive around the stomach and breasts. An elbow thrust back into the mugger's midsection may knock the wind out of her and give you time to run and yell for help.

A LIKELY STORY   After his last class of the day, Steven remained in school for a meeting of the recreation committee. It was almost 4 o'clock by the time he left the building. The rest of the students had gone home and just a few older boys were playing basketball in the schoolyard.

As Steven started to walk, his mind was wandering. He may have been thinking about the meeting in school or he may have been looking forward to the steak his mother was going to broil for supper. Whatever was on his mind, Steven wasn't thinking about being mugged. Because of this, he violated a basic rule—he was not alert. This mental lapse caused Steven to walk too close to the building. By doing this, he was an easy prey for the man who was hiding in the alley way at the edge of the school.

As Steven walked past the alley that led back to the playground, the man grabbed him from behind and put his right hand over Steven's mouth. The man held a knife with a 6-inch blade in his left hand. He placed this under Steven's chin and told him not to move.

Steven had been carrying some school books and a brief case. The moment he was grabbed, he dropped these—perhaps out of fright or perhaps to leave his hands free if he had to defend himself. Afterwards, he wasn't sure if this move was deliberate or not. But once the books were on the ground he noticed that his left hand was close to the mugger's groin. He knew he had a chance to hurt the mugger if this were absolutely necessary.

Steven's mouth was covered so he couldn't talk. All he could do was listen and take a deep breath to relax. He tried not to think about the cold edge of the knife that was pressing against his throat. Finally, the young man spoke. His voice was threatening but almost friendly. "Listen kid," he said, "hand over your money and you won't get hurt."

Steven's money was in his left front pocket. He moved his hand slowly from where it had been poised by the mugger's groin, reached into his pocket, and held the wallet up for the mugger. The knife remained at Steven's throat, but the mugger moved his other hand and slowly grabbed the wallet. Now that Steven's mouth was no longer covered, he was free to turn his head. He twisted it just slightly and got his first glimpse of the mugger. This occurred at the time that the mugger was taking his wallet. Steven recognized his assailant as a man of about 20, who was often seen loitering around the school grounds.

Steven's view of the mugger lasted for less than a second. The moment the man's focus shifted from the wallet to the victim, Steven was carefully looking in the other direction. "Now get out of here," he was ordered. Steven did what he was told. He left his school books on the ground, turned the corner, and ran.

This is not the end of the story. The boy was still faced with several decisions—should he tell his parents? Should he let someone know at school? What would he do if he happened to see the mugger again? Steven was not ready to go home alone, so he tried the school door and found that it was still open. Once inside, he was able to find the principal. Steven retold the whole story and the principal winced at the mention of the mugger's knife.

The boy was not in favor of calling the police, but the principal convinced him that this was important. Together they phoned the local precinct and received instructions to remain in the school. A squad car was dispatched to pick up the young victim, get his statement, and drive him home. Before the squad car parked in front of the school, it cruised through the area to see if anyone fitting the mugger's description was lingering near by.

As a result of this incident, the principal assigned male faculty members to patrol the schoolyard on days when there were after hours activities. When Steven had to stay late for a meeting, either a family member picked him up by car or he arranged to walk home with friends. For a few weeks after the mugging, police patrolled the area and questioned older youths who were in the vicinity for no apparent reason.

• • • There are a few subtle points in this story that are worth repeating. For example, when Steven started to walk home, he stayed close to the school building so he could remain in the shade. Had he been walking in the middle of the sidewalk or close to the curb, he might have been a more difficult target. The mugger might not have brandished a knife if he were away from the alley and in clear view of passers-by.

Steven did not have a chance to talk to the mugger, as I suggested earlier, but he did do something important. As soon as he was caught, he took a deep breath to keep from tightening up. Thus, while the mugger held him, he didn't squirm, fidget, or do anything that would cause the mugger to use his knife.

Another way that Steven showed good judgment was in resisting the temptation to get a good look at his assailant. Steven was able to recognize this man from just a casual glimpse out of the corner of his eye. But had the mugger caught Steven deliberately looking at him, the boy's life might have been in danger.

The action after the mugging is also important. Steven made the right decision when he went back to the school and notified the police. Another boy his age might have acted otherwise. Many youngsters are afraid to report a crime for fear the mugger or his friends may find them outside of school and get revenge. They also are afraid of the reaction of their parents. Either their fathers may overreact and go after the criminals themselves or their parents may blame them for not fighting to protect what is theirs. For these reasons, many crimes against juveniles go unreported. As a result, school-age children may be the most frequent victims of physical abuse and crime.

In other sections, I have asked you to put yourself in the place of the victim. For this story, I would like you to think as if you were the victim's parent. Would your own children have known what to do in this situation? Would they have confided in you if they were attacked? What precautions have you taken for your children's safety on the way to and from school?

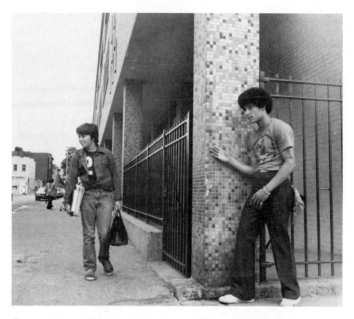

Steven is making two mistakes. He is not looking where he is going and he is walking too close to the building.

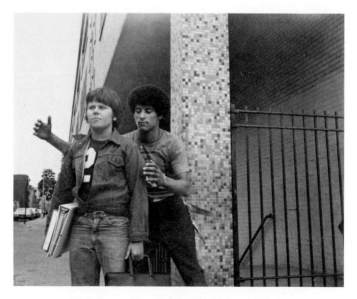

The mugger grabs Steven from behind.

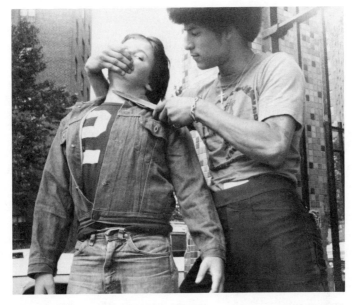

With a knife at his throat, Steven remains perfectly still so he does not panic the mugger. In the event that force is necessary, Steven's left hand is positioned near the mugger's groin.

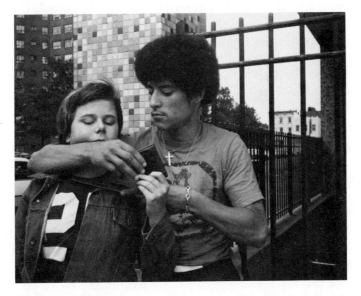

When the mugger asks for Steven's wallet, Steven gives it up without a fight.

Avoiding a Knife Thrust at Your Stomach

Mr. Silverio Mazzella was 71 when he attended one of my classes. It was an all day session in a senior citizen center in the South Bronx. When we broke for lunch, Mr. Mazzella went out to the street. There he was approached by a young man wielding a dagger. The man demanded a quarter. When Mr. Mazzella could not produce it, the young mugger aimed his knife at the older man's stomach. At this point, Mr. Mazzella relied on techniques that he had learned in the morning class. Within seconds, he had disabled the mugger and had taken away his weapon.

This may seem incredible, but it's true. After the incident, Mr. Mazzella returned to the senior citizen center and handed me the knife. I followed him outside and we found the mugger in a nearby doorway. He was still in pain.

Imagine my feeling! What I had taught that morning had saved a man's life. But how do you think Mr. Mazzella felt? He considered this one of his proudest moments—not because he had hurt a man, but because he had proved that he could still protect himself. At an age when many of his contemporaries were afraid to walk the street, Mr. Mazzella had become a hero.

I repeat this story in almost every lecture that I give. It reassures me that what I am teaching is worthwhile. It should also convince my listeners that despite their age or handicap, they are still capable of helping themselves.

The technique Mr. Mazzella used was a combination of three moves. The first move (assuming that the mugger has the knife in his right hand) is to stand on the balls of your feet and quickly pivot to the right. Thus, if you were facing 12 o'clock when you started, you would be pointing toward 3 o'clock in your final position. Stated in another way, if you were facing the mugger originally, your left side would be pointed at him after you completed your turn. Please note that your feet never leave the ground. You are not taking any steps. You are simply executing a right turn (or pivot) as you might do if you were in the army.

Since you are turning to avoid the path of the knife, you should not start to move until after the mugger begins his attack. Always keep your eye on the blade so you know where it's going. As the knife passes your side, hit the mugger's knife arm at the wrist with your left hand and push it away from your body. Then grab his arm so he cannot come back and stab you. This is the second step. Before going further, take time out and practice these two moves. Pivot to the right and forcefully raise your left hand. As you come to the later part of the turn, your left hand should be pushing and clutching an imaginary arm that is holding a knife. Do this over and over until the two moves—the pivot and the push—are perfectly synchronized.

When the mugger is trying to stab you, his eyes are focused on his knife. The hand that is empty is hanging uselessly at his side. Once you have avoided his thrust, the mugger is vulnerable to your attack. Keep your left hand on the mugger's knife arm, but turn your head so you are looking at the mugger's face instead of his weapon. As you turn your head, bring up your right hand and plunge your second and third fingers into the mugger's eyes.

These were the three moves that were used by Mr. Mazzella. He turned to the right, used his left hand to divert the course of the knife, and then used his right hand to strike a blow to the eyes. This caused the mugger to let go of his knife and drop his guard. Mr. Mazzella countered with further blows that left the mugger almost helpless. In this instance, he went beyond my instructions and improvised his own technique.

The method I have just described is used when there is no alternative. In the example above, the mugger wanted 25 cents and would not accept "no" as an answer. He was determined to stab and possibly kill the victim. Why didn't he succeed when he had the advantage of a deadly weapon and youth? The answer is that he didn't know what Mr. Mazzella was going to do. Mr. Mazzella used a small amount of force but he used it scientifically.

A LIKELY STORY When Dotty drove into a municipal parking lot, she passed a man who was seated on the trunk of a car. Dotty was too busy trying to park to pay much attention to this individual. There was a space next to where he was seated and Dotty swerved the car and parked it on her first try. As she got out of the car, she paused for a moment to lock the front door and to look at her reflection in the window. The man noticed this and he saw the large pocketbook that was hung over her shoulder and held loosely in her right hand.

As Dotty moved away from the car, the man walked quietly behind her. He was wearing sneakers and Dotty didn't hear him approach. Suddenly she saw someone pass her and she felt a tug on the strap of her pocketbook. The man had rushed by, had grabbed the front of the strap, and was trying to run away. Without thinking, Dotty held onto the bag and pulled back. She had all her shopping money inside and she didn't want to let it go.

The man turned to pulled harder and Dotty deliberately put her second hand on the strap of the bag. Now he was holding on with one hand and she was pulling with two. She seemed to have the advantage.

While Dotty's attention was riveted on the tug of war for the pocketbook, she noticed the man reach back with his right hand. A moment later, she saw something flash out of his back pocket. The man was still holding the strap in his left hand, but with his right he was aiming a knife at Dotty's middle.

At this point, Dotty was no longer concerned with the fight for the pocketbook. She let go with her left hand and poised herself for the mugger's attack. As he lunged forward, Dotty completely let go of the bag and twisted to the right to elude the blade.

When the knife thrust past her, Dotty hit the mugger's wrist with her left hand and pushed it further away from her body. As she did this, she grabbed the mugger's arm to keep him from pulling back the knife and stabbing again.

Now both of the mugger's hands were occupied. His right hand was holding the knife and his left hand was clutching the pocketbook. In a sense, the mugger was defenseless. While he was attacking, Dotty had been staring down at the knife. Now that she had avoided being stabbed, she looked up at the mugger's face. With two fingers extended on her right hand, she reached out and poked the mugger's eyes.

The mugger's head jolted back and he dropped the knife. Dotty did not stop to pick up the weapon or recover her pocketbook. She ran for the street to find a policeman.

• • • There are a few points in the story that are worth reviewing. First, Dotty was not sufficiently observant when she was parking the car. The presence of the man should have made her suspicious and caused her to park somewhere else.

Once her pocketbook was grabbed, Dotty's initial instinct was to hold on. Many women react in the same way. They resist the mugger by impulse rather than design. By doing this, they may risk their lives to save just a few dollars.

I try to combat this impulse in my classes by having my assistants walk through the audience and snatch pocketbooks. The women know in advance what's going to happen. They know that their belongings will be handed back to them. But even then, some people are reluctant to let go. You can see how strong the impulse is to protect personal property.

While Dotty made two mistakes that led her into danger, once she recognized the danger she acted flawlessly. She stopped thinking about the pocketbook and she concentrated on the knife. When she hit the mugger's arm, she used enough force to keep the knife from coming toward her. (This is important to remember because when some people practice this move, they make just a token gesture with their left hand. Merely touching the mugger's arm is not enough.) There was just a moment's lapse between the time that Dotty avoided the knife and the time she struck the mugger. A fast response here is essential.

Finally, after Dotty was free, she didn't stop to grab her pocketbook and she didn't try to get to her car. While the vehicle may seem like a good means of escape, she would have lost valuable time when she unlocked the door and started the ignition. Had the mugger recovered and followed her, she could have been trapped in her own automobile.

How would you react if something of yours was taken and the thief was trying to get away? Would you react the same way that Dotty did? How long would it take you to learn this technique so you could use it effectively? Do you think you are capable of fighting off an assailant with a knife?

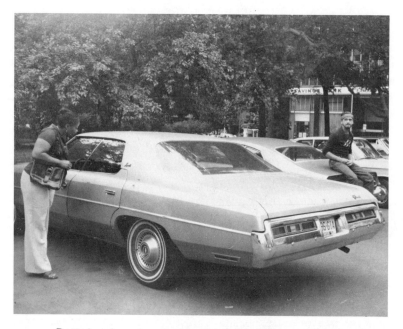

Dotty has been spotted by the man sitting on the car.

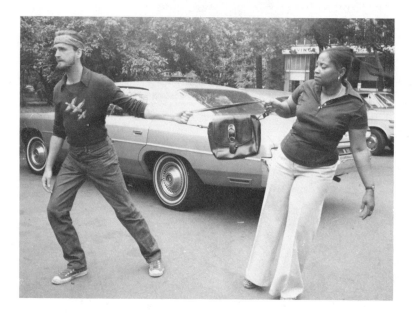

He grabs the strap of her pocketbook from behind and tries
to run off with her bag. Dotty instinctively holds on.

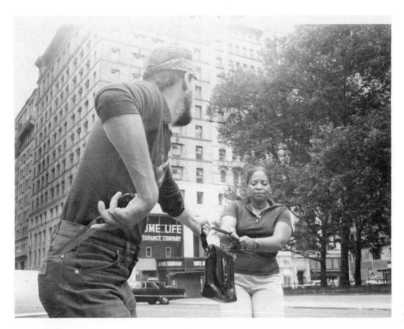

Dotty tightens her grip on the bag and the purse snatcher reaches for his knife.

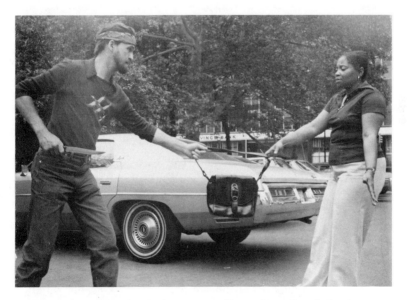

Realizing that she is in danger, Dotty lets go of the bag with her left hand.

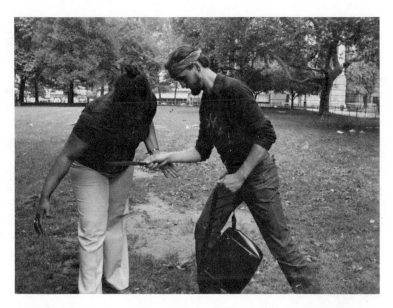

As the blade comes near her body, Dotty pivots to the right and hits the man's wrist with her left hand. By doing this, she forces the knife away from her body.

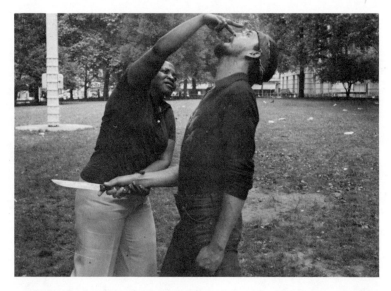

Dotty maintains a grip on the man's wrist. With her other hand, she pokes him in the eyes.

Applying the Wrist Throw

This technique is appropriate when you are attacked by a mugger with a knife. As the mugger thrusts his knife toward you, you should pivot to the right so that the blade misses your body. With your left hand, hit the mugger's arm near the wrist and push it off course. These are the same actions that were called for in the last section. What makes this technique different is the way you will use your right hand.

This time you *will not* use your right hand to poke the mugger's eyes, you will use it to disarm him. As the mugger's knife hand is driven away from your body, strike the back of his hand with your right palm. The direction of your blow should force the mugger's wrist back toward his own body. If the impact is sufficient, the mugger will feel considerable pain and may possibly drop the knife. But this is just the beginning.

Hold onto the back of his knife hand with your right hand. Reposition your left so that your two thumbs are together. Then force the mugger's wrist further back and then sideways and down. You can use this grip to lower the mugger to the ground, and, if you use enough pressure, you can sprain or break his wrist.

Note that as you hit the mugger with your right hand, you should cup your thumb and fingers. This will allow you to hold onto the back of his hand. Whatever you do, don't let go. Maintain your grip until you have completed the throw and the mugger has released the knife.

As you force the mugger's wrist down, you should change the position of your feet. When you were avoiding the thrust of the knife, your left hip was pointed at the mugger. Now you should pivot on your right foot and turn almost 90°. Thus you and the mugger will be practically facing in the same direction.

By twisting the mugger's wrist sideways and down, you will move him closer and closer to the ground. As the mugger's wrist is forced down, the rest of his body will follow. To gain more leverage you can step with your left foot in the direction he is being thrown.

When you have completed the throw, the mugger will be on his back with his knife hand raised slightly above him. (Note that you are still holding onto this hand.) If the knife was not jarred loose when you first hit his hand, the pressure on the mugger's wrist will cause his fingers to close around the handle. When this happens, you are still not safe. It may be necessary for you to kick the mugger in the face or the head.

These blows will have two effects. They will lessen the mugger's ability to fight back and they may loosen his grip around the knife. At this point, you can attempt to pry the knife out of the mugger's hand. Only two precautions are necessary. You must be careful to grab the knife by the handle and you should not spend too much time in trying to get it away. The longer you take, the more time the mugger has to recover. The effects of the wrist throw and your kicking may wear off and the mugger may regain the upper hand. If you cannot get hold of the knife immediately, start to run before the mugger is in condition to resume the attack.

In 1974, this throw was used by one of my former students— Horace Orton—to disarm an attacker. He describes the incident in the following letter. It is interesting to note that although Mr. Orton had not practiced this technique for some time, he was still able to execute it properly when his life was in danger.

Dear Liddon:

I think I would be remiss in my obligations somehow, if I did not write to express my deepest feelings in regard to a serious incident that happened on April 19th in my office. I will always be grateful for the day you started that judo-jujitsu class for Housing Authority employees in which I was given an opportunity to train in the martial arts, keep physically fit, and learn first aid. Who would ever suspect that after only one year of study that the training would save my life as much as four years later. Everything happened so quickly on that Friday afternoon. To this day, I can hardly believe it took place.

I was conversing with two female employees in my office and completing the day's work. It was nearly time to go home when we were interrupted by another employee who appeared at the door. He had a grievance about a personal matter which was not clearly stated. I realized that he had been drinking and invited him to return Monday when he would be in better shape. He was very persistent and I couldn't reason with him. Evidently, he was tired of talking because he whipped out a knife and snapped it open. My friend, a greater sense of danger I have never felt. That knife was all of ten inches long and at least an inch wide. I backed away from him slowly. I tried to give him time to think about what he was doing. I sensed the wall at my back. I was now trapped in a corner as this guy came on. I had absolutely no weapon with which to defend myself. You may not believe this, Liddon, but I really thought I was about to die.

This man, who was quite stocky, finally lunged at me. I saw a flash of pale steel coming at my neck. By sheer instinct I reacted. With a sudden burst of forced energy that swelled within my body, I gave a familiar yell that we had heard so many times in your class. To my own amazement, I leaped forward to meet his attack. I stopped the movement of the knife just two inches from my throat. With one hand, I gripped his wrist. With the other, I circled his body and threw him to the floor. I was now on top of my attacker. Still holding tight that knife hand—so it was outstretched and pinned to the floor by my left—I shifted my weight and brought my right fist to his Adam's apple, thereby forcing him to release the knife.

Through all of this the two brave women staff members never left me alone. Paulette, my secretary, called in a policeman who hand-cuffed the man when I released him. And Eva, our clerk, moved the knife quickly out of reach without thinking of her own safety.

I wish to thank you very much for the straightforward, no-nonsense way in which you conducted your class. It allowed us to learn and take seriously the art of defending ourselves against such attacks.

With warm regards,

HORACE L. ORTON

To be able to use the wrist throw, you should memorize and practice the following steps. (Assume that the mugger is holding the knife in his right hand.)

1. As the blade comes toward your body, pivot to the right so that your left hip is pointing toward the mugger. If the knife is aimed at your midsection, suck in your stomach so there is more clearance between your body and the knife.
2. While you are moving your body, keep your eye on the knife. As you turn, hit the mugger's wrist with your left hand and push the mugger's arm away from your body. Note that once you make contact with your left hand you do not let go.

3. Hit the back of the mugger's hand with your right hand. The force of this blow should drive the mugger's hand back so that his hand and forearm almost form a 'U.' When you slap the mugger's hand, your thumb and fingers should be ready to hang on. The force of this blow will often dislodge the weapon. If it does, do not dive for the knife. Continue with this technique.
4. Once you have a tight hold on the mugger's knife hand, place your left hand next to your right so that the thumbs are together and facing in the same direction. Start to bend the mugger's wrist back toward his body, then sideways and down.
5. As you begin step 4, pivot on your right foot so you are facing in the same direction as the mugger.
6. Take a step in this direction with your left foot and, as you do, use your wrist hold to throw the mugger to the ground.
7. Even as the mugger falls, hold onto his wrist. If he is still holding onto the knife, kick at his face and try to remove the weapon from his hand.

A LIKELY STORY   In the springtime, Mark liked to do his homework on a bench in the park. At first he found it hard to concentrate. But with practice he learned to pay attention to his work and was able to shut out everything else.

One afternoon Mark was doing an arithmetic problem and didn't notice a tall black man who had walked over to the bench. As Mark suddenly looked up, the man grabbed him by the collar and pointed a knife right at Mark's body. "You white S.O.B.," the man threatened, "I'm gonna carve my initials on your gut." With this remark, the man tried to plunge his knife into the pit of Mark's stomach.

As the knife came toward Mark's body, he reacted in three different ways at once. He turned quickly so that the center of his body was no longer exposed to the blade. At the same time, he lifted himself a few inches off the bench and moved further away from the thrust of the knife. By instinct, he inhaled deeply and pulled his stomach in as far as it would go.

The combination of these three moves would have prevented Mark from being stabbed on the first try—although the knife would have only missed him by about 1 inch. He would have been an easy target if the attacker had tried to stab him again. But Mark did more than just move out of the way.

At the same time he twisted his body, Mark hit the man's wrist with his left hand and then grabbed onto it and held it tight. He used this hold to guide the knife away from his body. With his right hand, he grabbed the back of the attacker's hand. He did this hard enough to force the man's hand back so it was almost at a right angle to the rest of his arm. The man felt a sharp twinge where his wrist was bent. This pain was spread over the back of his hand and almost reached the knuckles.

Mark had hit and grabbed the man's hand at the same time. Once he established this hold, he moved his left hand off of the man's wrist and firmly placed it next to his right so that his thumbs were side by side. The man's hand was still jammed back in a painful position. As Mark started to twist it to the side and down, he got off the bench to get better leverage. At this point, his body had turned 90° from its original position. His left hip was pointed at the bench.

He took one step forward, and as he did, his arms swung in an arc that ended when the attacker was lowered to the ground. The impact of this fall caused the knife to slip out of the man's hand. Mark saw the knife lying on the sidewalk and kicked it as hard as he could. It traveled about 15 feet. Then with one final twist of the man's wrist, Mark let go and headed for the street.

• • • Reading a book or doing homework outside is pleasant, but if there's any chance of danger it keeps you from being alert. Mark would have been safer if he had been sitting with a friend.

This story is an example of an attack that was unprovoked. Had the man not announced what he was going to do, he could have stabbed Mark before Mark had a chance to protect himself. This actually happens. Many victims have told me that they were hit or stabbed before they had a chance to surrender their money or use any type of self-protection. In these cases, the only way the victims could have avoided injury was by being especially alert before they were attacked.

Getting back to the technique, this is an effective means of dealing with an armed criminal. From reading this section, you have learned all the moves you will need to use the wrist throw. My question is, "Will you be willing to take the time to practice them?"

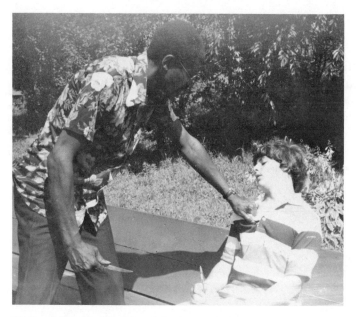

While doing his homework in the park, Mark is grabbed and threatened by a man with a knife.

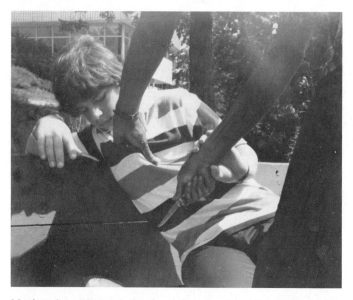

Mark twists his body to the left to avoid being stabbed. At the same time, he uses his left hand to change the direction of the blade.

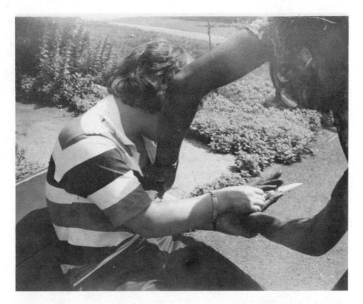

Mark holds on with his left hand and hits the back of the man's hand with his right.

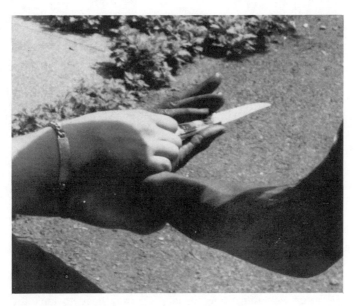

A close-up of the action in the previous figure.

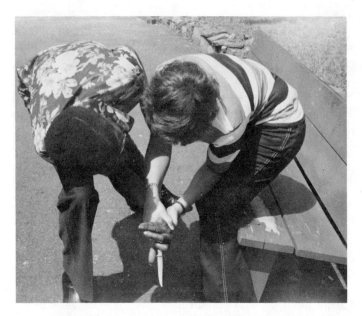

Mark twists the man's wrist sideways and down.

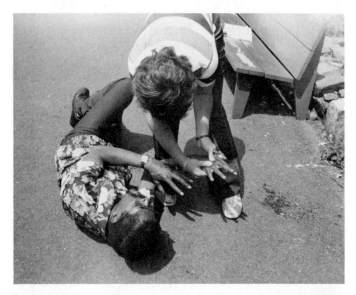

As he moves the attacker's arm closer to the ground, Mark steps forward with his left foot and completes the wrist throw. Mark will not release his grip until the attacker has dropped the knife. If necessary, he may have to kick the attacker's face and run.

Dealing with the Mugger Who Has a Gun

Having to defend yourself at gunpoint is the most difficult situation described in this book. There is no room for error. If you are going to resist, the only way to succeed is by getting the gun away from the mugger. I will show you two ways that this can be done when the gun is in range: one where the gun is pointed at your stomach and one where the gun is against your back. Before I describe these techniques, however, let me offer you some important advice.

If you are robbed by a criminal with a gun, you should not use force unless you think it is the only way that you can save your life. Before you try to resist, cooperate with the mugger in every way that he demands. If he wants your money, give it to him. If he asks you to disrobe, you may be embarrassed but do not hesitate. When you have met all of the mugger's demands, he will either leave or continue to hold you at gunpoint. If the gun is still on you and you think that the mugger may use it, you will have to try to escape.

First suppose that the mugger is in front of you and that his gun is flush against your stomach. Assume that this is a situation that is going to require the use of force. The mugger may first order you to raise your hands. You should do this, but only raise them slightly over your head. Do not hold them up straight.

Do not give the mugger any indication that you are going to resist. It is important to make him think that he is completely in command. Otherwise, if he feels the least bit threatened, he may be tempted to use his gun.

Another thing that you should not do is stare directly at the weapon. If the mugger sees you looking at his gun, it is not likely that you will catch him by surprise. What you will have to do is to keep your eyes fixed on his face, but to glance down slightly so you can notice the position of the gun and in which hand it is being held. Any forewarning of your actions can be fatal. It is important that you remain calm. Remember, if you try this move and lose, you lose completely.

If the mugger has the gun in his right hand, you should move your left foot slightly ahead of your right. In this position, you will be ready to perform the wrist throw that you learned in the last section.

Your first moves should be to step with your left foot and, at the same time, to twist your body to the right so that it is almost at a right angle to the mugger. As you do this, grab the mugger's wrist in your left hand and swing it in the direction in which you are moving. What you have accomplished is that you have repositioned the gun so that it is no longer pointed at your body. Even if the mugger pulls the trigger, you will not be hit.

Now use your right hand to bend the mugger's wrist and to force him down, as was shown in the last section. The important thing to remember is not to let go of his hand *until you have* the gun. In this situation, you are not safe unless you are holding the weapon. The reason for this is obvious. If you left the gun on the ground and you left the mugger in considerable pain—perhaps with a broken wrist—the mugger could still get to the gun and fire while you were trying to escape.

Thus, it is imperative that you never take your eyes off of the gun. If the mugger is still holding it when he is down, you may have to kick him in the neck or face to force him to let go, or you may have to strike the back of his elbow with your right fist, or maintain pressure on his wrist with your left hand until the pain forces him to let go of the weapon. Once he releases the gun, move *one hand* off of his wrist so you can gain possession of the weapon. It is important that you maintain the pressure on his wrist while you are reaching for the gun.

If you have forgotten how to apply the wrist throw, please go back and reread the previous section. The photographs in this section will also be helpful.

Now let us consider how you can protect yourself with a gun at your back. Once again the criminal has the advantage. The only good reason for resisting is to prevent him from using the gun. I would not use this technique just to save my money.

The sequence of events might be as follows: The criminal places his gun at your back and instructs you to raise your hands. You should do this, but do not keep your hands straight up. Raise them slightly over your head and keep your elbows bent. The criminal's next move is to slip your wallet out of your back pocket. Do not interfere. If he wants your money, let him have it.

At this point, the crime should be over. But suppose that you are still being threatened and suppose you feel that you are going to be shot. Under these circumstances, you will have to take action to disarm the mugger. There are two things that you will need to find out: Is the gun in range? And in which hand is it being held?

To get this information, turn your head slowly and look over your shoulder. Do not move your body, because the slightest movement may cause the mugger to use his gun. When you look back, do not look down. In this position, you will be able to see everything from the waist up. You can see how close the gun is to your back and you can see if the mugger is holding it in his left or right hand. Let us assume that he is holding it with his right.

Your first response will be a combination of two different moves. You will turn slightly more than 180° to the right. This means that if you start with your back to the mugger, after you have turned, your right hip will be pointing to the right of his body. At the same time that you are turning, straighten your right arm until your elbow is no longer bent. Lower that arm so that your hand is just a few inches above your hip and almost two feet away from it. (This distance will vary, depending on your height.) As you turn, the swing of your arm will hit the mugger between the wrist and the elbow. You will not stop at the moment you make contact, but will continue to turn and to drive the mugger's gun hand away from your body.

It is important to remember that this is not a two-part turn. Your body and arm must move at the same time. You cannot give the mugger any warning of what you are going to do. You must turn quickly so that you hit the mugger's arm with considerable force.

This is not the end of the technique. If you were to stop here, there would be nothing to keep the mugger from turning back and firing. Thus, as you hit the mugger's arm, you must be prepared to follow through and catch his wrist in your left hand. Once you have done this, your next move is to get your right hand on the back of the mugger's wrist and to start the wrist throw.

To diagram this procedure, let me describe your position in relation to the hours on a clock. When the holdup begins, you are facing "twelve." When you start to turn, your arm is extended and it is moving ahead of you. It strikes the mugger's arm at "six o'clock" and moves it past "six" so it is pointing away from your body.

You continue to turn and at, approximately, "eight o'clock" you catch the mugger's wrist in your left hand. At this point, you reverse directions. You add your right hand to the wrist hold you have on the mugger. Then you execute the wrist throw, as you move from right to left.

ABOUT THE PHOTOS   You have been provided with eight photographs that show you situations involving a mugger with a gun. In the first photo, the gun is pointed at the victim's head. You can see that it would be futile for him to try to resist. In this situation, the victim should make every effort to satisfy the mugger's wants.

You should also notice the difference in size between the victim and the mugger. The victim is almost a foot taller. Would this discourage the average criminal from attacking him? Most muggers would say "no." If they needed the money badly enough, they would attack anyone of any size. In this respect, the weapon is a great equalizer.

What do you think is the victim's reaction? Is it likely to be "frozen fright," as was described by Dr. Symonds at the beginning of this chapter? The person who posed for this picture had actually been robbed at gunpoint a few weeks earlier. He described his reaction as "controlled anger." He was furious at being victimized, but in this situation he could do nothing about it.

The second photo begins a new sequence. The gun is at the victim's stomach. Complying with the mugger's request, the victim has handed over his wallet.

If force is going to be necessary, this is a good time to begin. Notice that the mugger is looking at the wallet rather than at the victim. It may be that the mugger's gun hand can be grabbed before he has a chance to pull the trigger.

In the third photo, you see that the victim has been able to catch the mugger by surprise. With his left hand, he has grabbed the mugger's wrist and has forced the gun away from his body. This move must be made quickly so that the gun hand is away from the victim before the mugger can pull the trigger. In the position shown in the picture, you will notice that the gun is aimed away from the victim. Even if the mugger fires his weapon, the victim will not be shot. One reason that this is so is that the victim has changed the position of his body.

The fourth and fifth photos show the evolution of the wrist throw. Note that in the fourth picture the wrist has been turned so it is facing the mugger's body. The next move is to force the wrist to the left and then down.

To appreciate the pain involved in this procedure, put your own wrist in the same position as the mugger's. Then with your other hand push down on your knuckles until you can feel the pressure at the bend of your hand. Next twist your hand away from your body. What was your sensation? Do you think this would be an effective move if someone else was handling your wrist in the same way, but was exerting a greater force?

In pictures four and five, note how the victim is using his whole body—first to put extra pressure on the mugger's wrist and then to throw him off balance. In the fifth picture, you will see that the victim has taken a step to the left as he starts to move the mugger toward the ground.

The sixth photo introduces the third and final situation. The gun is at the victim's back. You can see that the victim has started to turn his head to look behind him. Note that the rest of his body has not moved.

In the next picture, the victim is in the middle of his turn. His arm has struck the gun hand and has swung it in a new direction. If the mugger were to pull the trigger, the victim would not be hit.

But that does not mean that the victim would be able to escape. He will not be safe until he has wrested the gun away from his attacker. To do this, he must continue to turn until he can grab the mugger's wrist with his left hand. This is the action that is shown in the final photograph. Once again, the victim is about to start the wrist throw. If you look at his eyes, you will see that he is carefully watching the gun. At no time can he let that gun be pointed at him.

• • • You have seen three different applications of the wrist throw: It is used to counter a knife thrust or to disarm a mugger who has a gun at your stomach or back. Do you remember how to use this technique? Try to walk through the movements with a partner, but do not use enough force to inflict any pain or injury. If you get lost as you are working through this sequence, look back to the photographs to refresh your memory.

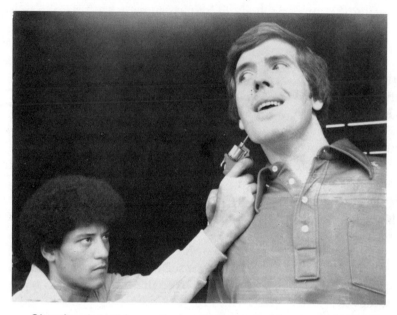

Situation 1. In this predicament, the use of force would be futile. The victim should make every effort to cooperate. If possible, he should try to verbally control the situation.

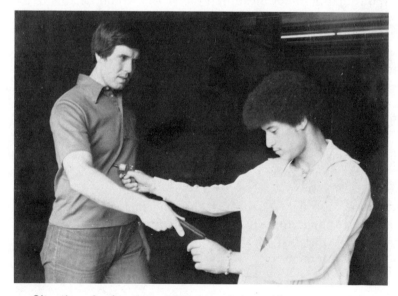

Situation 2. As the victim surrenders his money, the mugger's gaze is fixed on the wallet.

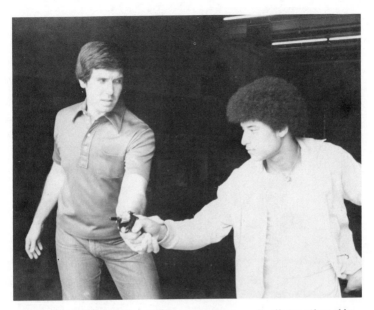

The victim takes advantage of the mugger's distraction. He hits the mugger's wrist with his left hand and forces the gun away from his body.

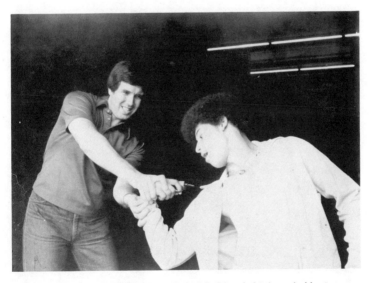

The victim establishes a grip with his right hand. He turns the wrist so that the mugger's fingers are pointing at his body.

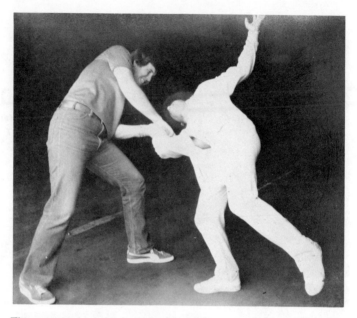

The mugger's wrist is twisted sideways and down. The victim steps forward with his left foot and throws the mugger off balance.

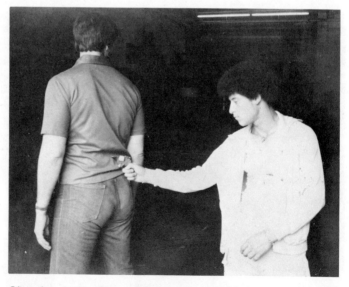

Situation 3. To disarm the mugger, the victim must turn his head slowly to see which hand is holding the gun. The rest of the victim's body should remain still.

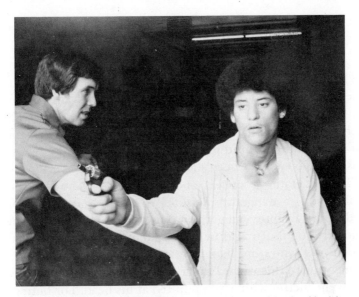

With his arm extended, the victim whirls suddenly. He hits the mugger's gun hand so that the weapon is no longer pointed at his body.

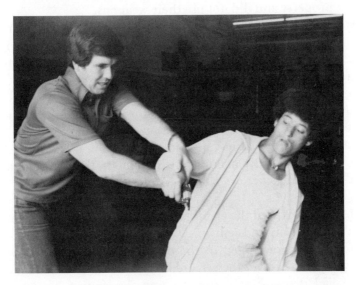

The victim continues to turn until he can grab the mugger's wrist with his left hand. Once this is accomplished, the victim reverses directions and places his right hand near his left. The next move is the wrist throw.

WHEN YOU THINK THAT YOU CAN'T USE FORCE

In the last chapter, I talked about how you could avoid danger without the use of force. To conclude this chapter, I want to return to that subject. There is a good reason for doing this. Each technique that I have presented has been followed by a story. In the story, the victim has used the technique to escape from the criminal. All of the victims in this book have been successful.

There is nothing unreal about this; the techniques actually work. But it is a dangerous mistake to think that what you have learned in this chapter can get you out of every situation. Sometimes the odds are too much against you. When this is the case, you must rely upon your wit rather than force.

I mentioned this when I described the victim with a knife at his throat or the victim with a gun pointed at his head. For both of these people, resistance would have been a mistake. Their only feasible option was to remain calm and to do nothing that would panic the mugger. In the stories, their behavior was rewarded. The muggers just took property and did not use their weapons.

An even better story was told to me by a secretary I met at New Rochelle High School. Her husband had been held up by two muggers as he had come off a train. One of the muggers had a gun against his head, and the other had a knife pressed against his throat. There was no sense in the victim struggling to get free.

The muggers helped themselves to his wallet and then started to remove his watch. At this point, the man spoke up politely. "That only has sentimental value," he said. "But you're certainly welcome to it if you want it." By making this statement, the man had accomplished three things:

1. He had convinced the criminals that the watch didn't have much value in dollars and cents.
2. He had acknowledged to the criminals that he was willing to give them whatever they wanted.
3. He had demonstrated that he was cooperative but calm. His poised demeanor set the tone for the rest of the encounter.

The end of the story is that the man was let go without being hurt. The criminals held onto his wallet, but they gave back his watch. In this case, good judgment was worth more than the knowledge of self-defense.

ABOUT THE PHOTOS　These pictures show a situation where the use of force would be futile. In the first photograph, a husband and wife are sitting on a park bench and reading a newspaper. You might argue that parks are dangerous and that the husband and wife are not being alert. You are probably right on both counts. But parks are made to be enjoyed and there is not much point in sitting outside if you are going to spend every minute looking for a mugger.

Does this sound like a contradiction? It isn't meant to be. Precautions are necessary, but once in a while we all let down our guard. It is impossible to protect ourselves against every crime. The only thing we can do is avoid situations where the risk is high.

The second photograph shows the couple surrounded by three criminals—two of them have weapons pointed at the man. There is no question that at this moment his life is in jeopardy.

If there is a key to his safety in this situation, it is not his strength or his cunning. Right now his life or death depends on the behavior of his wife. If she panics—if she starts to yell for help—either mugger may use his weapon.

• • • In this chapter, you have seen many examples of how you can use force to protect yourself. You have also seen a few situations where the use of force was not warranted. Only the victim can tell if the best course of action is to fight back or submit.

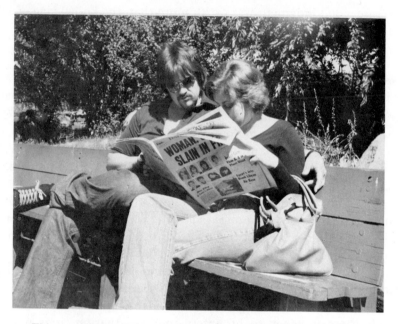

This couple is sitting in the park on a Saturday morning. Compare this scene with the one that follows.

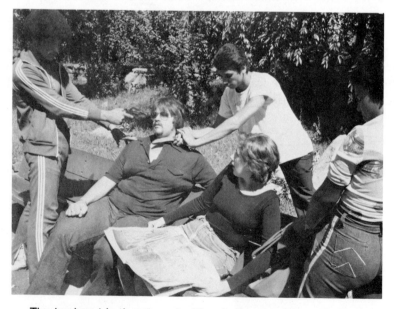

The husband is threatened with a knife and a gun. If either victim panics, the man will probably be killed.

130

5
Avoiding Rape

Most of what you have learned in the last two chapters will also apply to the crime of rape. For example, Chapter 3 suggested many ways of avoiding a mugger. These suggestions are also valid for avoiding rape. Your chances are always better if you are alert and if you are traveling with a friend.

In the same way, the techniques you learned in Chapter 4 can also be used to fight off a rapist. Some criminals will commit rape as an aftermath to robbery. When this is the case, you are in the same position that I described in the last chapter—the criminal has taken your money but he wants more. You will have to decide whether to resist or submit.

Many of the holds that we talked about in Chapter 4 can also be used by the would-be rapist. He may try one of the strangleholds to intimidate you. Or he may get you in one of the bear hugs to drag you off to a secluded place. If you have read the last chapter and have practiced the techniques, you will have a good opportunity to escape.

There are many parallels between mugging and rape. For this reason, I will approach the subject of rape in the same way that I presented the discussion of mugging. I will start with a description of the rapist, then suggest ways of preventing rape, and, finally, I will demonstrate a few techniques that can be used after the victim is on the ground.

(Before I begin let me point out that there are policemen and criminologists who have specialized in the study of rape. They have probed the motivations of the rapist and the anxieties of the victim. These students of rape are entitled to be called authorities.

My own experience is not that extensive. I have prepared this chapter from the information I have obtained from two types of sources: from my interviews with rapists and their victims and from my attendance at seminars devoted to rape. This chapter is not intended to be a detailed examination of the subject, but it should be a good introduction to this serious problem. In some places, you will find suggestions that you will not encounter elsewhere.)

PROFILE OF THE RAPIST

Dr. Symonds of the Karen Horney Institute divides all rapists into two categories: the rapist who commits the crime to satisfy a sexual urge and the predatory rapist. The second criminal resorts to rape as a means of abusing the victim.

When the motive is sexual satisfaction, the attacker may fantasize that the victim has been seduced rather than intimidated. With this in mind, he may talk to the victim during the sexual act and even give her clues that will indicate his identity. When the act is completed, the rapist may be contrite or may even try to make a date with the victim. Despite this behavior, it is a mistake to think that this type of criminal is not dangerous.

The predator may combine rape with other criminal acts. For example, he may take the victim's money and then to hurt her, he will abuse her sexually. For this person, rape is an act of violence rather than pleasure. He does not pretend that the victim is enjoying herself. He knows that she is terrified and this is his source of satisfaction.

Thus, there are two basic motives for committing the crime: One is sexual gratification and the other is the desire to physically dominate a member of the opposite sex. Many authorities feel that the second motive is more common. This might explain why young offenders make sexual attacks on senior citizens.

THE PREVENTION OF RAPE

In addition to the precautions suggested in Chapter 3, special care should be taken by women who live alone. It is a good idea not to alert a criminal to the fact that a woman is the only occupant of an apartment or a house. Thus, if a woman's name is listed in a directory of tenants, only her first initial—instead of her first name—should be given. The same rule applies to the listing of single women in the telephone book.

If you are confronted by a rapist, there is still a chance that you can escape without using force. This can be done if you are able to eliminate the first of the three elements of a crime—the desire to commit the crime. While you may not think that it is possible to demotivate a rapist, let me offer a few suggestions.

The rapist may not want to have physical contact with you if he thinks you have a contagious ailment. The venereal diseases are the ones that he will fear the most. But there are other illnesses that may keep him away. One woman told me that she convinced a would-be rapist that she was suffering from cancer and that he would catch it if he engaged her in sexual intercourse. It seems hard to believe, but this deception worked.

If you try this approach, you must persuade your attacker that he is proceeding at his own risk. In a sense, you are telling him that he can commit the crime if he is willing to suffer the consequences. The rapist may doubt your sincerity, but if he is the least bit unsure, he may leave you alone.

Another way to avoid danger is to convince your assailant that you really want to have sexual relations with him but that you prefer to have them in a more romantic setting. One woman told me that she invited a would-be rapist to her apartment. The pretense was that she wanted to shower first and slip into something more becoming. The man agreed to the later meeting. When he arrived at her apartment, he was met by the police and apprehended.

A third way to keep from being attacked is to make yourself less appealing to the rapist. You might tell him that you are in the first day of your menstrual period. Or you might try to make yourself vomit. This can be done by sticking one or two fingers down your throat.

Forcing yourself to regurgitate is unpleasant, but I believe that it will cause the rapist to back off. I have interviewed several sex offenders and all of them have indicated that they would not want to have intercourse with a woman who was vomiting.

The suggestions I have made are overlooked in most discussions of rape. I believe that if he is handled properly, the rapist can lose his desire to commit the crime—be it physical or sexual. When this is possible, it is the surest means of rape prevention.

FIGHTING BACK AGAINST THE RAPIST

As I mentioned before, the techniques you have already learned may help you if you are in danger of being raped. The question that I will raise now is, "When should you fight back?" Only you can provide the answer.

In the previous chapter, I suggested that you don't use force to protect property, but that you do fight back if your life or physical well-being is in danger. If you accept this suggestion as a guideline, how should you react if you are threatened with rape?

One consideration is that rape is often accompanied or followed by severe physical violence. The attacker may beat his victim to make her submissive or to enhance his sense of complete dominance. Once the act is completed, he may also use violence to discourage her from identifying him. Thus, the victim of rape may suffer more than just sexual abuse.

Even if the crime is limited to the penetration of the vagina, and the victim is not hurt physically, she still may suffer extreme mental anguish. While most victims eventually get over the effects of a physical injury, there are some women who never recover from the trauma of rape. Suppose that such a woman had an opportunity to relive the crime. Do you think that she would submit or, if she could use force effectively, would she try to fight back? My impression is that, given the know-how, she might try to resist.

To support this assumption, let me refer to two stories that demonstrate the impact of this crime. One woman I know was accosted on an elevator and dragged up to a rooftop by a would-be rapist. The assailant held her over the edge and threatened to drop her unless she promised not to resist. He then dragged her back onto the roof and began his assault. Even after this terrifying experience, she tried to fight back. She scratched at the man's face, but this did not help. She later told the investigating detective that the scratching seemed to excite the rapist rather than drive him away.

The important thing to note here is the victim's tremendous compulsion to avoid being raped—even when she was not trained in the use of force and when she knew that the price of resistance might be her life. Another experience that is worth repeating was related to me by a senior citizen I met at Coney Island General Hospital. She was attending one of my classes when she told me this story.

Two years earlier she had been attacked by a young man. When she had tried to resist, the man had laughed at her and said, "At your age, you need this." Try as she did, she was unable to fight him off.

To make the indignity even worse, when the man finally left he took all her clothes. She was forced to seek out help in the nude. As she told this story, her hands were shaking. It was clear that after two years she could still feel the shame and the fright of her terrible ordeal.

Now suppose that you were faced with the decision to fight or submit. You would have to consider the danger of being hurt and the possibility of being mentally scarred by your experience. You might decide to overlook these factors and not take any action. Your reason would be that you might not want to do anything that would antagonize the criminal and make him even more violent. The other alternative is to establish a guideline for the use of force. You might decide to resist if the criminal wants anything more than your personal property.

If you decide to use force, it is best that you try to escape early in the crime. There are three reasons for your wanting to get away quickly:

1. The sooner you escape, the less likely you are to be injured.
2. Your chances of getting away are better before the rapist is in position to commit the crime. Thus, if you are going to fight, you should do so before you are forced to the ground or before you are abducted to an out-of-the-way site.
3. The longer you remain inactive, the more difficult it will be for you to react. You will have to overcome your own inertia as well as your fear of antagonizing the criminal.

For these reasons, many authorities believe that you must react within the first 20 seconds. During this time, you can apply one of the methods that were presented in Chapter 4. If you are unable to react in time, you may be on your back before you have a chance to resist. In this case, you can employ one of the following techniques.

Getting Out of the Stranglehold
When You Are on the Ground

In the previous chapter, you learned how to escape from the stranglehold when both you and the attacker are standing. In this chapter, you will learn how to protect yourself when you and the strangler are in a different position. Assume that you have been wrestled to the ground and are lying on your back. The attacker is kneeling with his knees straddling your body. He is leaning forward and his hands are around your throat.

This scene occurs many times as a prelude to rape. The victim is choked by the rapist until she is either too weak or too terrified to resist. At this point, the rapist may rip open her clothes and commit the sexual act.

It is therefore important to escape while the rapist still has you in the stranglehold. The method you can use to get away is similar to the technique I described in the previous chapter. Once again, you can release the grip by hitting the strangler's elbows. But some other actions are required.

What you are trying to do is to get the strangler to let go and to get him off you. You can accomplish this by coordinating two moves. The first move is to bring your hands up behind the strangler's elbows and to hit his elbows with your hands moving toward you. This will cause his arms to bend and his grip to loosen. At the same time, the blows to the elbows will knock him off balance. Let me explain why this happens.

While the strangler is resting on his knees, he is leaning forward and supporting his weight with his arms. The harder he chokes you, the further forward he will lean and the more he will depend on his arms to keep him up. When you hit his elbows, his hands are lifted off your throat and his base of support is gone. Since he has been leaning forward, he will fall in that direction.

Only half of what you set out to do has been accomplished. You have caused the strangler to let go, but you haven't succeeded in getting him off you. If you only hit his elbows and pushed them forward, you would cause him to fall. But when he landed, you would still be underneath. Thus, there is a need for a second move. This must be executed at the same time that the rapist's elbows are hit.

If you think of what you have available, you will realize that your feet as well as your arms are free. I am going to suggest that you use one of your knees to push the strangler so that when he falls he will go over your head and not land on top of you.

While you are on the ground, bend one leg so that your knee is up in the air. You will use this leg for support and keep your other leg straight. At the time you hit the strangler's elbows and push them forward, bring your straight leg toward you so that your knee strikes the strangler's buttocks. To increase the impact of this blow, lean your weight on your other leg and arch your back slightly. The combination of the blow to the elbows and the knee to the buttocks will cause the strangler to sail over your head and land a few feet away from you.

What happens next depends on how you use your hands. If when you coordinate the two moves you hold onto the strangler's elbows, you will follow him through the air and land on top of him. By doing this, you have turned the tables in your favor. You can retaliate with a blow to the groin or eyes before the attacker is able to defend himself. The purpose of these blows is to incapacitate your assailant so you have an opportunity to get away.

The other course of action is to let the strangler sail over your head without holding onto his elbows. When you do this, you remain in place while the strangler lands a few feet away from you. To be able to escape, you have to get on your feet and start running before the strangler can catch you.

In my opinion, your chances are better if you land on top of the strangler, but even if you don't, you still have an advantage. The important thing is not to hesitate. If you stop to see where the strangler has landed, you will lose valuable time.

If my class is held in a gymnasium, or if there is a chance to take the class outdoors, I like to let people try this technique. Usually, one of my assistants or I will play the attacker and one of the smaller students will be the victim. The victim is usually surprised at how easily a bigger person can be thrown. But not everyone is convinced. Some people will suspect that the strangler is being too cooperative. When this is suggested, I will select someone from the class and let him get on top of the victim. The new strangler will also be thrown and will be quick to testify that the technique really works.

Before you read the story that accompanies this technique, please make sure that you remember the two key movements.

1. Bring your hands up behind the strangler's elbows and hit his elbows with your palms.
2. Keep one leg bent and one leg straight. When you hit the strangler's elbows, bend your straight leg so that your knee strikes his buttocks.

Remember that both blows should be forceful. Just making contact is not enough.

A LIKELY STORY   While many senior citizens are concerned about crime, there are some older women who walk the streets with great confidence. They feel that if they are confronted by a criminal, he will not abuse them out of respect for their age. At the same time, they think that because of their advanced years they will not be subject to sexual attacks. Unfortunately, experience has proved that neither assumption is entirely accurate. In the story that follows, Mrs. Kay is an example of a woman who felt unduly secure.

She had lived in the same neighborhood since the day she was married. Over the years, the neighborhood had changed and the crime rate had steeply risen. Most of Mrs. Kay's friends had moved, but she and her husband had staunchly refused to give up their apartment. As she explained, "No bunch of young rowdies are going to force me out of the place where I live."

Mrs. Kay had retired a few years earlier, but she still remained active. She participated in community affairs and kept in contact with several friends. On Wednesday afternoons, she would meet one of her friends in a local park and the two ladies would walk together and then go for a late lunch.

On this particular Wednesday, she waited for her friend by a clump of hedges in the center of the park. As she waited, a man who had been concealed in the bushes behind her stepped out and boldly grabbed her around the neck. With his arm curled around her throat, he lowered her slowly to the ground and then pounced on top of her.

Mrs. Kay had not heard the man come up behind her. When she felt herself choking and was aware of the pounding in her chest, she thought she was having a heart attack—or possibly a stroke. Her body went limp and she offered no resistance as she was lowered to the ground. It was not until she was on her back and the attacker was crouched over her that she realized what was going on.

Once she saw the man and she understood his motives, she knew that she had to fight back. His knees were on either side of her body and he was bent forward with his hands tightly clutched around her throat. Mrs. Kay's first reaction was to grab his hands and to try to pull them off her. But she was not able to do this. She was matching strength against strength and the would-be rapist had the advantage.

After this failed, she reached up to the man's chest and tried to lift him so his hands would come off her throat. But once again she was not successful. Each of these moves lasted for only a second. Mrs.

Kay was acting on instinct. When she had first been lowered to the ground, she had almost blacked out. She had imagined that she was being lowered onto a stretcher and was about to be taken away. When her back had struck the ground and she had seen the man above her, she had come to. Her immediate reaction was to resist; but in the first few seconds she was not thinking clearly.

Mrs. Kay knew how to escape from this position. Before she had retired, her employer had offered a class in self-defense. Mrs. Kay had attended every session and had learned several techniques, although she never thought that she would have to use them. As she now looked at the would-be rapist, she remembered how she could get him off her body.

She was still being choked. Her feeble attempts at resistance had caused the man to press harder and to lean further forward. Mrs. Kay noticed this as she raised her hands directly behind the strangler's elbows. At the same time that she positioned her hands, she bent her left leg slightly so that her knee was a few inches above the ground. Her other leg was lying flat but was ready to strike.

There was no reason to hesitate. Mrs. Kay had been watching the strangler's arms so she would be sure to hit them squarely. As soon as she was ready, she slapped the strangler's elbows from behind. The blows knocked him forward and Mrs. Kay grabbed onto his elbows and continued to move him over her head. He no longer had her in the stranglehold.

The elbow strikes were accompanied by a blow from her right knee that hit the strangler squarely in the buttocks. Mrs. Kay did not have to watch this happening; she knew if she brought her leg straight toward her, she couldn't miss. To add to the impact, she shifted her weight to her left leg and arched her back slightly. The combination of the blows from her hands and knees propelled the strangler through the air. He landed a few feet away from his original position with Mrs. Kay still clutching his elbows. While in flight, the two bodies had turned so that the woman was almost on top of the man.

When Mrs. Kay hit the ground, she released her grip with her right hand and struck the attacker in the groin. As he rolled in pain, Mrs. Kay got up and hurried out of the park.

Once she was on the street, she found a policeman. At his suggestion, she was taken to the hospital for a precautionary examination. There she was found to be in good condition, but the doctor recommended that she rest at home for at least 48 hours before she resumed her normal routine.

The friend whom Mrs. Kay had been expecting arrived a few minutes late. When Mrs. Kay was not at their customary meeting spot, the friend called her home and got no response. She tried the number a few more times and then returned home.

In the evening, Mrs. Kay called her and said that she had become sick on the way to the park. As a result, she had taken a taxi to the hospital so she could be examined.

• • • In introducing this story, I said that Mrs. Kay felt unduly secure. Do you think it was an unnecessary risk for her to wait alone in the park? Remember the neighborhood had an increasing crime rate.

If your employer were to offer a course in self-protection, would you want to join?

When Mrs. Kay's friend could not reach her at home, do you think she should have notified the police?

Was Mrs. Kay right in not alarming her friend or should she have told her the truth? Perhaps she was too embarrassed to relate the incident to anyone else.

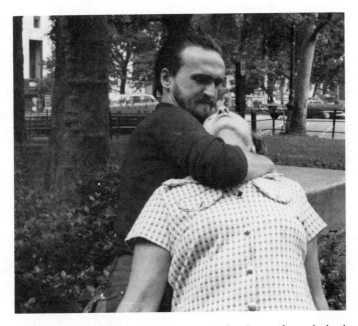

A few seconds before this scene took place, the criminal was concealed in the bushes.

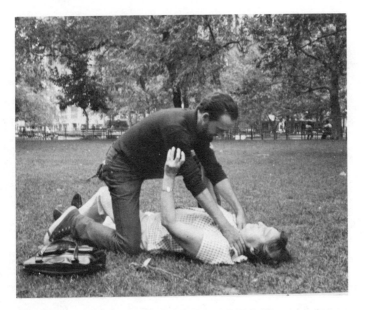

Mrs. Kay has been wrestled to the ground. The man is trying to choke her into submission.

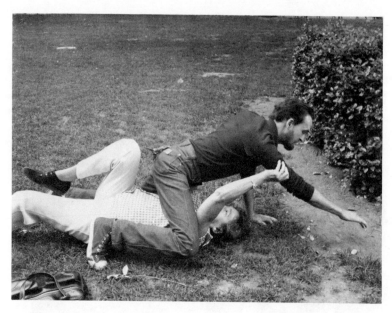

Mrs. Kay hits the man's elbows from behind and drives them forward. With her right knee she strikes the man in the buttocks and pushes him over her head.

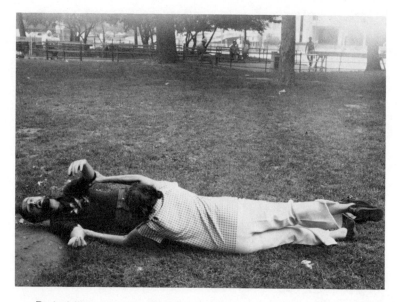

By holding onto the attacker's elbows, Mrs. Kay follows him through the air and lands almost on top of him.

Another Way to Escape from the Rapist

This technique is designed for the situation where you are on your back and the rapist is covering your mouth with one or both of his hands. You cannot yell for help. But you do have the use of your arms and legs. This is one way you can use them to get free.

Assume that the rapist is kneeling with one knee on either side of your body. He is bent forward and, to some extent, he is supporting his weight with both of his hands. You know that his hands are the only things that are holding you down. If you can get them off your mouth and throat, you should be able to squirm free and the rapist will be thrown off balance.

Now the question is how to move the rapist's hands. The common tendency is to grab him by the wrists and to try to pull his arms to the left or right. This approach is seldom successful. Even if the victim is able to move the rapist's hands, she is still on her back and not in position to get away.

A better approach is to use your body as well as your hands. First roll to your left and strike the inside of your attacker's right arm with your open right hand. The blow should be struck close to his wrist. Continue to roll past the point of contact so that the rapist's arm is pushed away from your face. By moving your entire body, you have all your weight behind you. The rapist's arm is displaced much easier than if you tried to move it with just your hand.

As soon as the man's right arm is clear of your body, reverse directions and roll back to your right. Use your left hand to hit his other arm. As you do this, continue to turn until your back is facing up. In this position, you can crawl out of the mugger's reach. Once you are a few feet away, you can get up and start to run.

To use this method successfully, you will have to move fast. When you knock the attacker's arms off of your body, he will probably topple forward and use his hands to break the fall. This keeps him from landing on top of you. It also gives you a few seconds to get away. The reason that you have to move quickly is that the rapist has not been disabled. There is nothing to prevent him from getting up and chasing after you.

If this is the situation, are you in greater danger after you have broken away? Is your resistance likely to make the rapist more vio-

lent? The answer to both questions could be "yes." But my viewpoint is that you are always safer when you are free. There is a
chance that you won't be caught and a possibility that if you are
caught you can use another technique to re-escape.

Another argument for trying to get away is that you know the
attacker is not after your property, he is after you. At the least, you
will be subjected to the indignity and mental anguish of rape and
you may be seriously injured. If you escape and are recaptured, how
much worse can your fate be?

The important things to remember about this technique are:
(1) You will be aiming at the inside of the mugger's arm; (2) you
must turn your body at the same time you move your arms; (3) each
hand hits the arm that is further away; and (4) after contact is made
for the first time, you must roll back in the opposite direction and hit
the other arm.

THE SECOND HALF OF A STORY   Judy had been attacked by surprise
and was stretched out on the ground. A would-be rapist was kneeling
over her. He had one hand on her throat and his other hand was
covering her mouth. Judy's entire body was free, but when she tried
to get up the two hands restrained her.

The attacker was leaning forward and was contemplating his
next move. Before he could act further, Judy raised her right side off
the ground. She rolled to the left and reached for the inside of the
attacker's arm—the arm that was further away from her right hand.
The force of her whole body turning helped her push the attacker's
arm until it was away from her mouth and no longer over her body.
At this point, the man was slightly off balance. His weight had
shifted to his right.

Without pause, Judy turned back in the other direction and hit
the attacker's other arm. She knocked it clear of her throat. The man
had been supporting his weight on his hands. As he lost his grip on
Judy's throat and mouth, he started to fall forward. He reached out
with both hands to keep from hitting the ground.

As the attacker was losing his balance, Judy was starting to get
away. She had originally been lying on her back. When she forced
the arm away from her mouth, she was turning left and her right hip
was pointed up. When she came back to dislodge the other arm, she
was turning right with her left hip up. She continued to roll until

she was in a crawling position. At this point, she slipped through the rapist's outstretched arms and slithered along the ground for about 10 feet. With this slight head start, she was able to get up and run before the rapist could catch her.

• • • Do you think that Judy made a mistake by trying to get away? If the man had been able to catch her, would she have been in greater danger?

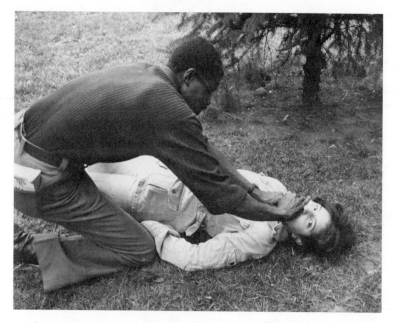

Judy's mouth is covered so she can't yell. The rapist's other hand is pressing down on her throat.

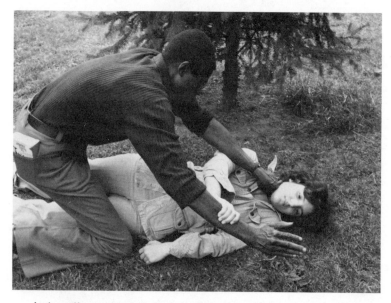

Judy rolls to the left and pushes the man's right hand off her mouth.

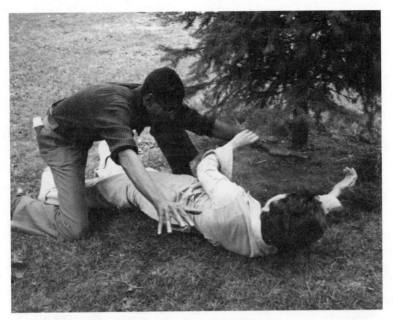

Only partially free, Judy rolls in the other direction and hits the mugger's left arm.

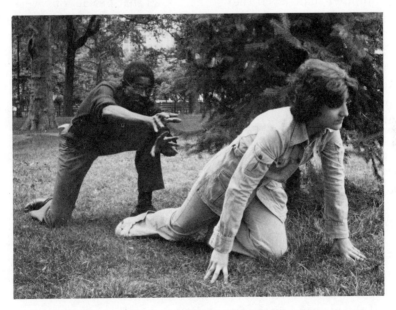

After the last move, the rapist is off balance. Judy crawls through his outstretched arms and starts to get away.

GETTING HELP AFTER THE CRIME

When a woman is raped, she is not the only one who suffers. In a sense, the entire family is victimized. While the woman bears the greatest burden, her husband and family also feel the effects.

From my experience as a police officer, I have seen rape damage a happy family relationship. The woman who has been violated may become withdrawn. Without reason, she may feel partially responsible for the crime. And for a long time after the crime, she may be haunted by the shame and humiliation of her ordeal.

For these reasons, the woman who is raped may feel uncomfortable and embarrassed in the presence of her husband. At the same time, she is desperately in need of her husband's support. It is tragic to note that in many cases the husband will be unable to give her what she needs. He will find it almost impossible to offer her his tenderness and reassurance.

There is an explanation for the husband's behavior. He may find it difficult to accept the idea that his wife has had intercourse with another man—even though he knows that her actions were not voluntary. He may also be hurt by the change in his wife's attitude. And he may feel that she is making him suffer for something he didn't do. As a result, the husband's role may change from comforter to accuser. He may intimate that his wife provoked the attack and that she actually enjoyed it. By doing this, he is reinforcing her worst fears and doubts. This causes the situation to grow worse instead of better.

For the husband to be able to help, he must recognize that his wife has been the victim of a crime. He may hold her responsible for the crime occurring, but this is probably unfair. In almost all cases, the victim makes no attempt to attract the attention or arouse the sexual desires of the rapist. Most victims of rape are attacked by surprise.

It would also be unfair for the husband to suspect his wife of not trying hard enough to resist. Many women do fight back, but to no avail. Many women are terrified by their attacker and are convinced that they will be killed if they do not cooperate.

If the husband or the family cannot offer enough support, there are outside agencies that may be able to help. Throughout the country there are many rape crisis centers. These organizations will counsel the victim and assure her that she is not to blame for what has happened. They will also speak to members of the family and help them to understand the crime and the dilemma of the victim. The rape crisis center will also inform victims of their rights under the law and will channel victims to the proper authorities in the police.

Many victims will hesitate to turn to the police for assistance. They may fear retaliation from the rapist, but they are probably more afraid that they will be badgered by the person who interviews them. At one time, this fear was well-grounded. Not long ago, a policeman might challenge several points in a woman's story. He might handle the interview indelicately and might suggest to the woman that a crime had not been committed because she had either enticed the rapist or had been a willing participant in the sexual act. Because of this approach, many women who reported a crime to the police felt that they had been abused.

Due, in part, to the actions of several women's groups, most police departments have come a long way in their treatment of victims. For example, most of the larger cities have sex crime analysis units. These units are notified of all sexual crimes and are specially prepared to work with the victims. When a woman who has been raped is referred to one of these units, she is usually interviewed by a policewoman. This spares the victim from having to explain the incident to a member of the opposite sex.

Even if a woman is questioned by a regular policeman—not a member of a special unit—she can anticipate that she will be treated with tact and respect. The old-fashioned police approach to rape has been generally abandoned. Every member of the force has been trained so they will know how to respond to the woman who has been sexually abused.

Despite this progress, many women are still timid about reporting a rape to the police. Their hesitancy is understandable, but it is hoped that these women will try to work with the police so that the rapist may be stopped before he attacks another person.

Outside Agencies

I have already mentioned the work being done by agencies outside of the police department. One such organization is New York Women Against Rape. This is a volunteer group that depends on public contributions for its existence. A brief description of the group and its philosophy is presented in the following extract:

> In 1973, New York Women Against Rape was founded as a result of the dramatic increase in the number of reported rapes in both New York City and the nation. We wanted to offer support to victims who often had no one to turn to. Since then, we have counseled over 1,600 rape victims and their loved ones on our weeknight hot line and/or in person. We have also participated in community outreach through the media and public speaking. It has always been our ideology that being informed about the myths and facts of rape alleviates the emotional trauma suffered by the victim of a sexual assault. Furthermore, a systematic program of community education would result in a decrease in crimes of sexual violence.
>
> The first fact that one must keep in mind is that rape is violence, not sex. There is no usual type of rape victim. Ages can range from 2 to 92. The woman can be beautiful or unattractive, a moral saint or disorderly, and may represent any race, creed or color. Our clients have been raped at any and all hours of the day and night and in a wide variety of places—home, work, school, or on the street.
>
> Just as there is no average rape victim, there is no typical rapist. Some correspond to the image of the sex-crazed maniac, but the majority seem to resemble the average man-on-the-street. In some instances, women know their assailants, but this does not mean that the woman has not been raped. The sexual attack still results in rape crisis trauma, which is a term that describes the guilt, anguish, fear, and mental confusion that can last for years. Such trauma interferes in the daily living habits and relationships of the victim. She generally feels as if she has lost control over her whole life.
>
> Most rape victims resolve to take some action or precautions to prevent another attack. Most would probably agree that if they were in a similar life-threatening situation, they would size up the assailant, their own abilities, and the environment around them and then react according to their instincts.
>
> If you are suspicious of someone, don't be afraid to be rude. Women especially have been taught to be "nice" in any and all circumstances. Trust is to the advantage of the rapist whose goal is to isolate the woman. "Street harassment" is a term that all women know from experience. Some rapists use this public verbal abuse as a warm-up for rape. They enjoy the fear and embarassment that it produces.

The attacker likes an easy victim. An alert appearance doesn't make a woman look easy enough. Alertness can be conveyed by an erect posture, with the head held high and a walk that indicates that you have a definite place to go. When you get to that place, check to see if there is someone ready to follow you in.

New York Women Against Rape is an organization that is solely dependent upon the time of a volunteer staff and whatever donations it can get. We have been unable to concentrate as much as we would like to on rape prevention and education. But we believe that our outreach program and other programs throughout the country may discourage possible rapists and may encourage informed confidence on the part of women.

VICKIE ANNE O'DOUGHERTY
and ALEXANDRA BONFANTE WARREN
Rape crisis counselors with New York Women Against Rape.

6
Self-Protection for Youngsters

The information presented in the first five chapters pertains to all age groups. For example, both young and old people can follow the methods of avoiding crime that were discussed in Chapter 3. The techniques demonstrated in Chapters 4 and 5 can be applied by adolescents or senior citizens. This chapter, however, discusses problems that primarily concern young people. These problems can be divided into two types: (1) the youngster's fear of being robbed or molested in the school or in the vicinity of the school, and (2) the youngster's fear of being subjected to violence where robbery is not the motive.

I have written this chapter because I believe that teenagers and preteens are victimized and abused more than any other age groups in our population. The actual number of crimes against young people cannot be accurately measured. This is because a large percentage of these crimes are not reported to the police. Why victimized youngsters remain silent will be explained later. The important thing to recognize now is that crimes against the younger generation are extremely widespread.

While this discussion is limited to one age group, I am aware of the fact that people of all ages are concerned. When I talk about children at a meeting of adults, people throughout the audience perk up. There are always parents and grandparents, or aunts and uncles, who are interested in the welfare of our young. If you have a child or grandchild in school—or if there is any youngster that you care about—I think you will find the following presentation worthwhile.

ROBBERIES IN AND AROUND THE SCHOOL

Although most school-age youngsters do not carry large sums of money, boys and girls in school are often mugged. These crimes may be committed by persons outside the school community who loiter in the area of the school or they may be committed by gangs of youths who attend the school. In either case, the perpetrators are not likely to be identified for a few reasons.

1. Students fear retaliation. If they accuse one member of a gang, they are afraid that other members will find out and get revenge. If the gang members attend the same school as the victim, he or she will have to face them daily and may be subjected to daily threats and daily abuse. There is also the possibility that the person who commits the crime will go unpunished. This happens often with youthful offenders. When this is the case, the person who has made the complaint will surely be afraid of retribution.
2. Students don't like to turn in a fellow student. Youngsters are taught from their first day in kindergarten that nobody likes a tattletale. While mugging is a serious crime, some students will hesitate to report another youngster. There seems to be an unwritten code of behavior that says "Rather than squeal, it is better to grin and bear it." The trouble is when you choose the latter alternative, the mugger is free to victimize someone else.
3. Students don't like to tell their parents that they've been robbed. This reaction may seem peculiar, but it can be explained in several ways. The youngster may fear that his parents will blame him for not fighting back. Or he may be afraid that his father will try to find the mugger and get revenge. Or, what is more likely, he may expect his parents to come to school and report the incident to his principal or teacher. The student may consider the last course of action very embarrassing—especially if the mother rather than the father reports the crime. Teenagers like to feel that they are mature; this feeling is undermined if their parents come to school and speak up for them. Another drawback is that once the crime is reported, the student is left in the predicament that I described in item (1). Rather than face any of these possibilities, many youngsters will come home and try to hide the fact that they've been robbed.

One of the places in school where youngsters are likely to be victimized is the bathroom. This may be a hangout for kids who are cutting class, for students who want to sneak a smoke—cigarette or marijuana—or for outsiders who have entered the school to commit a crime. The bathroom stalls provide a cover for all of these individuals. In many schools, the boys' and girls' bathrooms are considered danger zones.

This situation is sometimes so severe that youngsters will avoid going to the bathroom until they have left school. Of course, this type of abstinence is unhealthy. If an area in a school has a reputation for crime, the best way to reduce crime in that area is to have it patrolled by an adult monitor. If possible, the school should hire security personnel. If the budget will not tolerate this, the principal can ask off-duty faculty members to tour the troublespots. For the example I mentioned, students can help one another by traveling to the bathroom in pairs. When this is done, one student goes into the bathroom while the other waits in the doorway. If the first student encounters any trouble, the person in the doorway can run out and get help.

The same type of awareness that I stressed in Chapter 3 is necessary in this situation. Before students enter the bathroom, they should look inside to make sure that there is no one there who doesn't belong. If students suspect danger, they should go back to their classroom and notify their teacher.

A LIKELY STORY   When school was in session, the doors of Metropolitan Junior High School (name is fictitious) were never locked. As a result, it was not hard for people who were not connected with the school to wander in and out. On a few occasions, these unwelcome visitors had robbed one of the students. This was the situation when Mark entered the bathroom on the second floor. He saw three men who were too old to be students and he knew that they were not members of the faculty. He realized that these people did not belong in the building. His best course of action would have been to turn around and walk out of the bathroom. But Mark was afraid that if he did this, the men would know that he suspected them and they would come after him. Rather than take this chance, Mark tried to pretend that he didn't notice anything unusual. He walked up to the sink and at this point he was attacked.

One man came up behind him and pushed his head into the basin and turned on the water. While Mark's head was submerged, a second man went through his pockets and removed his wallet. The third man stood at the bathroom door to watch for outsiders. In a matter of seconds, the crime was over and the men were heading for the staircase. Mark had never seen them before and had not had a long enough glance at any of them to make a good identification.

• • • Mark's decision to stay in the bathroom got him in trouble. He would have been safer in the halls, where he might have been seen by other students and members of the faculty. Once Mark was attacked, he had no real opportunity to resist. His only choice was to give up his money and hope that he would not be hurt.

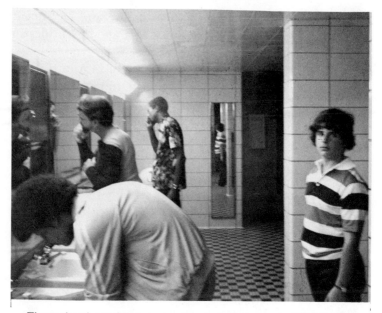

The school washroom can be a danger zone. When Mark saw three people who didn't belong, he should have left the washroom immediately.

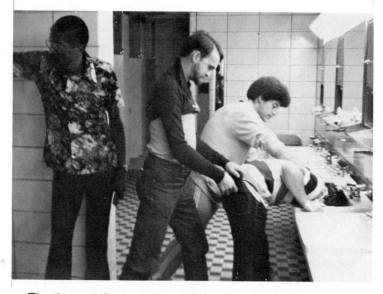

The three outlaws work in unison. One forces Mark's head under the faucet. Another goes through his pockets and the third looks for members of the faculty.

Other Danger Zones in the School

While school bathrooms are notorious as a site of crime, they are not the only places in a school where crime may occur. Students may be mugged in any area that is not well supervised. Examples of other danger zones may be the lunchroom, the staircase, or the schoolyard.

Students are more susceptible to robbery or attack if they remain in the school area after classes are over. Schoolyards are often a hangout for older members of gangs. If schools allow their yards to be used for recreation after hours. the school should provide some type of adult supervision.

Where youngsters remain in school for extracurricular activities, it is preferable to have these students leave the school building in a group. As with adults, students are more likely to be mugged when they are by themselves. If parents are particularly worried about students who have activities after school, the parents can arrange to transport these students in car pools.

Who Victimizes the Young?

As most students do not carry large sums of money, they are not attractive targets for the professional mugger—the criminal who carefully selects his victims. While some youngsters are mugged by adults—as in the story that you just read—most crimes against the young are committed by people who are young themselves. Their motive for committing these crimes may be to get more money but it may also be to establish a reputation with the members of their gang. When this is the case, the young mugger may be considered a status seeker. (This type of criminal was described in Chapter 2.)

Let me tell you a story about a group of status seekers who robbed a high school student of his lunch money. The student was approached by a small gang and surrendered his $2.00 without an argument. Even though he cooperated, he was soon informed by the gang leader that they were going to beat him up. The victim had no opportunity to use force. He was greatly outnumbered and had to rely on his wit. Rather than beg to be let go—which would have made a beating inevitable—the victim tried a practical approach. He said to the gang, "You guys know that you can beat me up, but if you leave me alone I'll bring you $5.00 tomorrow." This appealed to the members of the gang and they let him go free.

The victim was one of my sons. When I heard what had happened, I wanted to go after the other boys to make sure that they didn't get away with this crime. But my wife convinced me to speak to them instead. I went to the gang without identifying myself as a police officer. I told them that they had robbed my son once and I wouldn't complain, but if they tried to take his money again, I would surely report them to the authorities. A few days later, my son was approached by a few members of the gang. They didn't threaten him again; they gave back his money.

I cannot say whether my son's actions or my own would be successful in every case. My reason for repeating this story is to give you a glimpse at the psychology of the gang. They took $2.00 from their victim. Split several ways, this was hardly a profitable venture—especially when the victim was able to identify them and would see them the next day in school. Their reason for wanting to beat the victim was not to intimidate him—he had already cooperated—but to solidify their own self-image. This was part of the role of being a tough guy in the school. Finally, after the crime was committed, the gang members returned the money without being asked. This probably demonstrates that all of them have good qualities in addition to the traits that led them to commit the crime. It also shows that to these muggers the money that they stole was not very important. The idea of committing the crime was what was really attractive. In many ways, this gang is typical of the people who victimize the young.

VIOLENCE FOR ITS OWN SAKE

While youngsters may be concerned about muggings that take place around their school, this is not their primary source of worry. Many youngsters are afraid that at some time they will encounter a hostile group of youths and that they will be pressured into a fight. When I spoke to students, I was surprised at how many of them had experienced this type of fear. What I basically heard was that kids were afraid when traveling to and from school. They were wary when they were in a new neighborhood or in any territory where they considered themselves outsiders.

When I asked students to elaborate on who they were afraid of, their descriptions varied. Youngsters living in middle-class suburbs would talk about cliques of two or three tough individuals. Teenagers who lived in the rougher neighborhoods of the city would admit that they were afraid of the organized gangs and their arsenal of weapons. In both cases, the descriptions pointed to a tight-knit body of youths. This body might be aggressive toward any youngster who was not part of the group. By being aggressive, I mean that the clique or gang would antagonize a youngster or provoke him until he felt obligated to fight. Once a fight ensued, the youngster might have a chance to win. But what is more likely is that he would be beaten and injured by one or more people.

The purpose of this violence would not be to rob the victim or to gain revenge for some previous abuse—although retaliation is a powerful motive in fights that break out between gangs. The real reason behind the type of fighting that I have described is that many youngsters are looking to develop an image. They want to convince their friends that they are both manly and tough. To do this, they try to pick a fight and beat up an outsider.

Avoiding This Type of Danger

When I questioned youngsters, most of them felt that they could avoid this type of violence, but to do so would involve a loss of face. The attitude of most was that they had too much pride to back down from a bully or from a group of bullies. The explanation that I heard over and over was that the youngsters had to maintain their image.

This concept of image—which affects the abused as well as the abuser—to me seems out of proportion. It is important to have a good opinion of yourself and to be admired and respected by your friends. This is what a good image is all about. But there may be ways to avoid a fight and still protect that image. Let me offer you an example.

Assume that you are walking down the street and your path is blocked by a group of teenage boys. As you approach them, you can tell that they are not going to move. Thus, you are left with a few choices. You can turn around and go back. But this might encourage them to come after you. You can try to walk around the group, but sometimes they will spread out to prevent you from doing this. Another choice is to keep walking and not give any ground. When you do this, you are hoping that someone on the other side will move out of the way and let you pass. But this is not what usually happens. What is more likely is that you will bump into one of the other youths. The youngster will shove you back and this bumping will lead to a fight.

None of these choices are ideal. What I would suggest is that you continue to walk in the same direction. But when you get within range look at the person in front of you and say "Excuse me." This gives the person an opportunity to move out of the way without being embarrassed in front of his friends. You are not challenging him, you are asking him politely. I have discussed this situation with many gang members, and almost all of them have said that if someone approached them in this way, they would not respond by fighting.

Unfortunately, the type of behavior I am suggesting is difficult for many youngsters. In this situation, they can't seem to utter the words "Excuse me," "I'm sorry," or any other statement that might seem to imply weakness. Once again the culprit is the word "image." Being even mildly apologetic does not fit with the role that many youngsters want to play. Where this is the case, I would hope that parents, guidance counselors, or older brothers and sisters could reason with the youngsters. A teenager has almost an entire lifetime to build an image. It would be a shame to jeopardize that lifetime because of one incident that wasn't very important.

WHAT ADULTS CAN DO TO HELP

Many parents have told me that they feel like helpless bystanders. While they see their children every day, they are not aware of their children's fears and they are not aware of what they, as parents, can do to make their children safer from violence and crime. Here are a few suggestions.

Children should be taught about crime as soon as they are allowed out of the house by themselves. The idea of this instruction is not to terrify them or to make them distrustful, but to train them to take the proper precautions. Most parents have found that if children develop a habit at an early age that habit will stay with them through adolescence. Thus, it is important for children to be exposed to crime instruction while they are still young.

As children get older, it is more difficult for parents to stay in touch with them. But it is well worth the effort. If your children can make you aware of their fears, you may have a chance to help them—either by offering your advice or by discreetly intervening at the school to get more adult supervision. But many children have difficulty communicating these fears. They consider being afraid the same as being a coward. And all children have been taught to be brave.

To prevent losing contact for this reason, parents—and fathers especially—should be careful not to make their children feel guilty for not standing up to youth gangs or older youths. If children expect this type of reaction from their parents, they will not be likely to confide in them. When this type of communication is lost, parents have no chance to offer their assistance.

Children will also conceal things from their parents if they expect their parents to overreact. I mentioned this when I spoke about the youngsters who were afraid that their fathers would actively seek revenge or that their parents would come to school and make a scene. Youngsters will not be open with their parents if they expect that their parents' reaction will strike them as being dangerous or embarrassing.

Where it is possible—and this may be a tall order—parents should make children aware of adult values. Everyone admires the person who is strong and brave, but it also takes a courageous person to say "Excuse me" or "I'm sorry." If your children are not capable of this response, they are left with one less way to avoid a fight. It would be helpful if you could teach them that being polite is a sign of maturity and not a sign of weakness.

Finally, you can make your children less susceptible to danger and crime if you keep careful track of their activities. This does not mean snooping, but it does mean establishing certain agreed-upon rules. You, yourself, can be a good judge of what these rules should be. One activity that *I* would suggest should be prohibited is hitch-hiking. This is a matter of great concern to the police. Hitch-hiking is against the law and in the event of an accident the hitch-hiker is not covered by insurance. Even more important is the fact that youngsters who hitch-hike are vulnerable to many types of crime.

They can be robbed, beaten, sexually molested, or kidnapped. Rather than risk any one of these experiences, youngsters should make a practice of not accepting rides from strangers.

• • • This has been a very brief discussion of a very serious problem. The adult will recognize that just a few answers are contained in this chapter. The important thing to remember is that youngsters are often abused and they need our help.

7

What You Can Do at Home

In the first chapter, I stressed the importance of preparation and called it "your key to safety." In this chapter, I will show you how you can spend just a few minutes a week to reinforce what you have learned. I will also suggest a few precautions that you can take now so you are prepared for an emergency.

In my judgment this chapter is as important as any of the others. Reading this book may have been your first step toward protecting yourself against the dangers of crime. But it is just a beginning. Without practice and review, the ideas that you learned in Chapters 3 and 4 will be of little value. The next section will explain why.

WHY PRACTICE IS NECESSARY

Think back to a movie that you saw last month. How much of it can you remember? Can you describe the entire plot from beginning to end? The chances are you can't. You may have been interested in the film and you devoted your entire evening to it, but probably not much of the movie has stayed with you. For a more emphatic example of how much we forget, think back to a subject that you studied in school. Do you still remember it today? What are the chances that you could take an examination in this subject and still pass?

The point is that when we stop talking about something or we stop using it, we tend to forget it. This is one reason why practice is important. To help you retain what you have learned, I will suggest a few drills that you can do at home. I have also provided some short quizzes (in Chapter 8). It would be a good idea if you try these quizzes every few months. If your scores start to go down, you know it is time to go back to the book and review.

There are other reasons why practice is important. One strong argument in its favor is that if you are mugged and you decide to resist, a very fast reaction is needed. There will not be much time for you to select a technique. You will have to know what you are going to do almost immediately.

Once you choose a method of escape, it will have to be executed quickly or you are not likely to succeed. Any hesitation on your part will give the mugger an opportunity to defend himself. Or, if he has been hurt, it will give him a chance to recover and to regain the advantage.

When you read about the techniques in Chapters 4 and 5, you saw them demonstrated step by step. This approach makes them easier to learn. But when you need these techniques, they cannot be applied as a series of isolated movements with pauses in between. They must be executed as one continuous motion. This is only possible with practice.

There is one other explanation for my stressing the need for continuous drill. People often say to me, "Sure, we can use these techniques in class, but if we were on the street and our lives were in danger could we use them then?" There is no question that being mugged is a very frightening experience. We don't know how we will respond to a mugger until we are actually his victim. But the advantage of practice is that it prepares us for that situation. By acting out a mugging—or by even thinking about it—we eliminate a part of the initial shock if we are ever confronted by a dangerous criminal.

This aspect of drill is utilized by the armed services. Thus, in basic training, new soldiers are exposed to gunfire. While the soldiers do not face any real danger during this exercise, the noise of the weapons acquaints them with some of the terrors of war. It is hoped that from this experience, the soldiers will be less likely to panic when they are involved in their first real battle.

THE AMOUNT OF PRACTICE REQUIRED

One of the selling points of my system is that the techniques are easy to learn. When I wrote the first draft of this manuscript I entitled it "KISS—Keep It Short and Simple." Those words were a guide to me in choosing methods of resistance. If I considered a method that required more than a few simple movements, I left it out of the book and replaced it with something easier to use.

As a result of this policy, long practice sessions are not needed. I usually suggest just three ten-minute sessions a week. After students are acquainted with the system, they can cut down to just one minute a day. It is never a good idea to stop practice entirely. There is always some danger of forgetting or becoming rusty.

Practice sessions are not strenuous. So there is no reason why elderly people or people with physical ailments cannot participate. If because of your health ten minutes seems too long, you can increase the number of weekly practice sessions but cut down on their duration. If you do this, you may want to limit one session to the techniques to be used against the unarmed mugger and devote the next session to practicing techniques to be used against the mugger who is armed. In this way, you are not likely to leave anything out.

Once you decide that you are going to practice, make up a schedule for yourself. If you plan to practice on Monday, Wednesday, and Friday, mark these days on a calendar and check them off as you complete each drill. At the end of the week, look at the calendar and see if you have reviewed the techniques as often as you planned. If you haven't—and this is not unusual—schedule extra sessions for the following week.

THE METHODS OF PRACTICE

The first thing to do is to skim through Chapters 4 and 5 and to make a list of the techniques you want to practice. Next to each technique in your list, enter the page numbers where it is discussed in the book. In this way, if you forget something, you can go back to the book and look it up. I would suggest that you keep the list and the book together and that you have both of them in the room where you intend to practice. Refer to the list during every drill, so that you don't accidentally omit any one of the techniques. Every few weeks, it is a good idea to rewrite the list and change its sequence. If you can perform the techniques in any order, you know that you have really learned them well.

Practicing by Yourself

If you have no one available to act as a mugger, you can practice by yourself with the help of a coat, a hanger, and a hook. The coat will represent the attacker. It should be kept on a hanger so it retains the shape of a body. An overcoat can be used, but you will find a raincoat much lighter and easier to work with.

To begin your drill, get a picture hook and screw it into the wall at about eye level. Then hang the coat and hanger on this hook. When you do this, the shoulders of the coat are slightly higher than your own. Thus you are pretending that your attacker is slightly taller than you are.

Now look at your list to see which situation you are going to re-create. Suppose it is the knife thrust. You will walk over to the coat and use the right sleeve to represent the mugger's arm. (This is demonstrated in the first page of photographs.) Hold onto the sleeve the same way you would hold the mugger's arm if you had just avoided the thrust of his knife. Your body should be at a right angle to the coat—remember you have just pivoted to escape the blade. Where should your eyes be? Right! You should be looking past the edge of the sleeve to where the mugger would be holding the knife.

Now you are in position for the next move. You are going to strike the mugger in the eyes. Do you let go of his knife hand? Not a chance! Hold onto the sleeve with your left hand and with your right hand poke the wall a few inches above the top of the coat.

Now let's consider a different situation. Suppose you are caught in the mugger's yoke—a type of stranglehold that is applied from behind. To simulate this hold, stand with your back against the coat and wrap the sleeve around your neck (see the second page of photographs). When you feel yourself being choked, what is the first thing you should do? I hope you said that you should turn your head so that your chin is pointing over the mugger's elbow. When you do this, you give yourself more room to breathe and you reduce the chance of strangulation. In the photograph, you can see that the girl has moved her head into this position.

If you study the photograph, you can see that the person who is practicing has made a mistake. She is twisting her head in the proper way, but she is holding the sleeve in the *wrong* hand. Because she has used her left hand and not her right, her left hand is not available for practicing the next two moves—the thumb to the eyes and the shifting of the body followed by the squeeze of the mugger's testicles. When you practice by yourself, watch out for this type of mistake. Try to re-create as much of a technique as you can. Remember that a technique is not finished until you have actually escaped.

Working with a coat is a good memory drill. You might say that instead of this, you could reread the instructions for each technique or you could say them over in your mind. But reading or saying is not the same as doing. Even though a coat is lifeless and offers no resistance, it gives you a chance to put the techniques into action. If you practice a method often enough with a coat, you may be able to use it (the technique) when you are attacked by a real person.

I have shown only two techniques that you can practice by yourself. But you can use a coat to work on all the other methods shown in this book. Or you can use it to invent methods of your own.

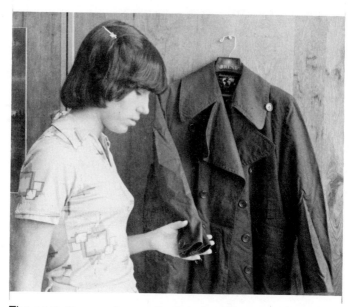

The coat represents an attacker. In this scene, the young lady is practicing the technique to be used when the mugger is thrusting a knife at your stomach.

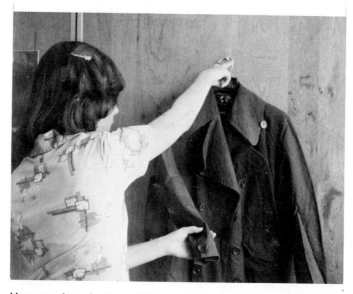

Use your imagination. With her left hand, she has forced the knife away from her body. With her right hand, she jabs the mugger in the eyes.

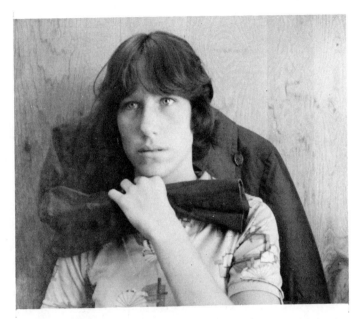

Using the coat, the model pretends that she is caught in the mugger's yoke.

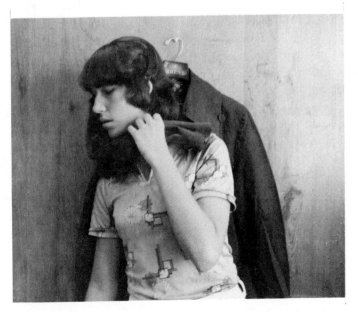

To avoid strangulation, she twists her head to the place where the mugger's arm would be bent.

Practicing with a Partner

When two people practice together, they can take turns playing the roles of the victim and the mugger. When this is the case, it is up to the mugger to consult the list and select the situation. The victim should not know ahead of time what hold the mugger is going to apply.

As the victim works his way out of a hold, the mugger should also function as an observer. After the escape is complete, the mugger should be able to tell the victim if he has used the technique correctly. Thus, in any re-enactment, both parties are concentrating on the technique and both parties should be learning.

The person who takes the part of the mugger may not be sure of how to apply a certain hold. If this happens, the mugger can take time out to look at the pictures in the book. This will not be time consuming if your list of techniques is complete with page numbers.

Proper restraint is very important when you are practicing with another person. Never make contact with the eyes or the genitals. If this is part of the technique, move your hand or foot to the proper position and announce what you are going to do. It is also important to go easy when you practice the pinch or one of the throws. The idea is not to injure your partner.

You can practice escapes from an armed mugger by giving your partner a rubber knife or a water pistol. When you practice with these devices, there is a way of testing just how well you are doing. Fill the water pistol with water—or, if the mugger is using a knife, make sure that the tip of the blade is wet. Then practice the technique. What you don't want to feel while you are practicing is the spray of the water pistol or the wet edge of the knife.

The photographs show a senior citizen practicing an escape with a gun at her stomach. She is hitting the mugger's wrist with her left hand and twisting her body out of the line of fire. If in the second picture the mugger were to squeeze the trigger, his elderly victim would still be dry.

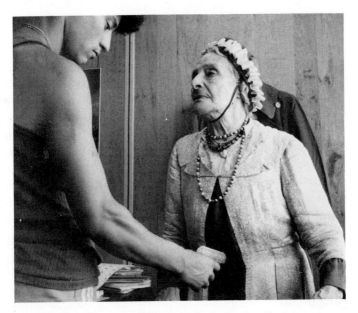

The use of a water pistol will let you know if you can use this technique successfully.

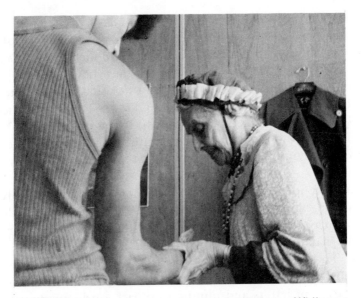

Pivot and push the gunman's hand out of the way. While you are doing this, the gunman will squeeze the trigger. If you get wet, you know you have failed.

Playing Identity Games

In talking about practice, I have only mentioned the rehearsing of techniques. But there is another skill that can benefit from training. This skill is your ability to observe a mugger and be able to identify him afterwards. If you are able to develop this capacity, you can give a good description of an assailant to the police and there is a better chance that he will be caught.

To practice identification at home, thumb through a magazine and stop at a color photo of a person. Look at the picture for five seconds and then turn the page. How much can you remember about the person? You should at least be able to answer the following questions.

1. Male or female?
2. Young or old?
3. Short or tall? (This may be hard to determine from a photo.)
4. Slim or heavy?
5. Race?

After you have done this a few times, you should be able to remember additional information. This would include items such as hair color and hair length (although they both are subject to change), color and style of clothing (as I mentioned in Chapter 3, it is a good idea to concentrate on pants and shoes), and any noticeable scars. Do not try to remember too much. If you do, you are likely to forget some of the most important details. Once you can describe a picture of an individual, try looking at pictures of two or more people.

Another identity game that you can play at home involves license plates. Sometimes you will not get a look at a criminal's face, but you may see him or an accomplice drive away in a car. It is possible that the criminal can be traced if you can remember his license. To practice this type of identification, buy a package of index cards and give a few of them to a friend. Ask him to write a combination of letters and numbers on each card—six characters in all. At the bottom of each card, he should print the name of a state. When your friend is ready, ask him to show you a card for three seconds and then turn it over. Your job will be to write down the license number and the state. You may find that you do not have enough time to remember everything. But three seconds is a realistic interval. In that amount of time, a car cruising at 25 miles per hour could travel 130 feet. At that distance, the printing on its license plate would not be legible.

OTHER TYPES OF PREPARATION

There are other things that you can do now to prepare yourself before a crime occurs. Some of these precautions were mentioned in Chapter 3. But I will describe them again, so you can include them in your list of things to be done at home.

Perhaps the best way to start is to make sure that your home is secure. Check your front door to make sure that it has a sturdy lock and a lock guard. It should also have a peephole, so you can see a caller without opening the door. Make a habit of checking all the windows before you leave the house. The best prevention system in the world will not keep a burglar out if a window is left open.

If you are a woman living by yourself, you will have to take a few extra precautions. Make sure that just your first initial and not your first name is listed in the phone book. If you live in an apartment building and there is a directory on the main floor, make sure that just your first initial is used.

Next to the phone, you should keep a list of important numbers. These should include the phone numbers of two close neighbors, of the police department, and the fire department. If you need help in a hurry, it is better to have these numbers available than to have to get them from a phone book or from the information operator.

As suggested earlier, if you live in an apartment building and you use the laundry room, you should make arrangements to do your laundry with a friend. You should also make a schedule of when other tenants do their laundry, so you will have a good idea of when the laundry room is likely to be occupied. This is important because your friend may not always be available.

Before going out, be sure you have a dime or a quarter. Either one can be used in a payphone if you need help.

One of the worst things about having a wallet stolen is that there is so much work to be done in replacing important items such as licenses and credit cards. You will find that this job will be simplified if you have made photostat copies of all your important papers. These copies cannot be used in place of the originals. But the photostats will give you all the information you need when it is time to apply for replacements.

People who receive social security checks may want to arrange to have these checks mailed to their bank instead of their home. This will eliminate the danger of the check being stolen out of the mail box. It will also eliminate the more serious danger of the check being forcibly taken from you on the way to the bank.

Men who want to take extra precautions can purchase a money belt. These are still available at some clothing stores and will hold from 5 to 15 dollars. There are some people who carry whistles or noisemakers as attention getters. The idea is to use these if you are in danger of being attacked. I do not recommend the whistle because it can be used against you—it can be shoved down your throat. The noisemaker does not have this disadvantage. However, it will only get you help if people understand why it is being used. If you want to try one of these devices, the time to get it is now. Do not wait until after you are mugged.

Some women like to carry what I call "pocketbook weapons." These are everyday items that are small enough to fit in the pocketbook and can be used to hurt an attacker. Examples of these items are a nail file, a safety pin, hair spray, and a sharp pointed comb. The danger in relying on these weapons is that the mugger may be able to get them away from you and use them himself. But if you think that these weapons are worthwhile, you should put them in your pocketbook before you forget.

If you count the suggestions I have made, you will find that I have listed 10 things that you may want to do at home. It is possible that you can add to this list. The important thing is to start working on these projects before this book is put back on the bookshelf.

THE CHECKLIST

The following checklist has important questions about your neighborhood. Please write down your answers and keep a record of them. If there is a question that you can't answer, try to find the necessary information as soon as possible. Add this little bit of research to your list of things to be done at home.

1. What is the address (street and avenue) of your local police department?

2. What is the address of the nearest fire department?

3. At what time and on what corners can you find a policeman?

4. What gas stations in your neighborhood stay open on Sunday?

5. What stores or restaurants are open late in the evening?

6. Where are there outdoor payphones in your neighborhood?

7. What are the busiest streets in the vicinity of your home? Where is the nearest fire alarm?

8. What danger zones are close to your home? Are there places that are hangouts for gangs or that have bad reputations for crime?

9. If you have children in school, what route do they take home?

10. When people in your family do their routine shopping, what stores do they go to and along what streets do they travel?

8
Self-Evaluation

The purpose of this chapter is not to measure your intelligence but to let you see how much of the material you have retained. Please take each test and make a note of your score. As I mentioned in the last chapter, it would be a good idea to continue to take these tests at three-month intervals. If you do this and you see that your scores are going down, it may be a signal that you should go back to the book and review the key chapters.

TEST 1: AVOIDING DANGER

Write down or memorize your response to each question. Then check your work against the answer section and see how many questions you have answered correctly.

1. Of these three groups which is the most susceptible to crime: individuals who travel by themselves, women, or senior citizens?
2. Name three signals that will tell an experienced mugger that you are carrying something valuable.
3. List two ways to carry a pocketbook that make it an easy target for the purse snatcher.
4. Men will sometimes carry their wallet in a front pocket. Why is this a good idea?
5. Muggers sometimes hide in doorways or behind parked cars. What is a good way to detect a concealed mugger?
6. If you are on the street and you think that a mugger is following you, how can you test him by crossing the street?
7. If you are being followed by a mugger on the street, list at least two things that you may have available for getting help.
8. If you are being chased by a person in a car, in what direction should you run?

9. If you are a pedestrian and somebody in a car stops and asks you for directions, what is the one precaution that you should take?

10. Assume that you have driven home and that a car has followed you home and has pulled up behind you. What should you do?

11. You have gone to a shopping center at night. What is probably the safest place to park?

12. You are on the elevator and you are sure that you are going to be mugged. Your decision is to react. What is the first thing that you should do?

13. Suppose that you have entered an apartment building and you hear an elevator door starting to close. Why shouldn't you run to catch the elevator?

14. What is a dangerous mistake that some people make when they are getting their mail?

15. When John Resident returns to his home, he sees signs that someone has broken in. Mr. Resident enters cautiously and calls the police. Why is this a mistake?

16. List two things that you can do when you go out to make a burglar think that somebody is still in the house.

17. A salesman rings your doorbell and asks to come in. How can you check that he is legitimate?

18. A man in plain clothes rings your doorbell and says that he is a policeman. What is a safe way to verify this?

19. You are on a subway car with one other person. You suspect that the other passenger is going to mug you. Without using force, what can you do?

20. If you are trying to remember what a mugger is wearing, on what articles of clothing should you concentrate?

21. You are aware of a mugging taking place outside of your apartment. You want to get help, but you have no phone. How can you get assistance?

22. Someone is being mugged outside your apartment. You call the police and let them know what is happening. What else can you do to help the victim?

23. You are the witness to an escape from a crime. You do not see the criminal's face, but you see him leave in his car. What three things should you be able to tell the police? (All three pertain to the car.)

24. In Chapter 3, I suggested that if a mugger is holding you at knife-point, you speak to him in a very quiet voice. Why might this be a good idea?

25. Why should you always have a dime or quarter with you when you go out?

Answers to Test 1

See how your answers compare with the responses that follow. If you are not satisfied with what you remember, you may want to turn back to Chapter 3 and skim through it one more time.

(1) My records show that the lone individual is the person who is most susceptible to crime.   (2) The professional mugger will know that you are carrying something valuable if you keep looking around, patting your wallet, or clutching your pocketbook very tight.   (3) A pocketbook that is held by the strap is an easy target for the purse snatcher. Another mistake is to hold the pocketbook with the flap facing away from the body.   (4) When you keep your wallet in your front pocket, you can keep your hand on your wallet without looking conspicuous. (5) You can sometimes spot a mugger in a doorway or behind a parked car by noticing his feet. These often protrude beyond his cover.

(6) If you think that someone is following you on the street, cross the street and then cross back. If the person is after you, he will cross both times.   (7) To get help on the street, you can yell, look for a store or payphone, or sound a fire alarm.   (8) Run in the direction opposite to that in which the car is moving. This way the driver will have to stop and turn around so he can catch up with you.   (9) You can give directions to a driver, but do not approach the car.   (10) If you think that the car that is parked behind you has followed you, stay in your own car with the doors locked. If you get in trouble, start to honk your horn.

(11) When you drive to a shopping center at night, I suggest that you leave your car near a floodlight. This makes the car easy to find and it illuminates the area around the car.   (12) If you are on the elevator and you know you are in danger, your first reaction should be to press several buttons.   (13) When you run to catch an elevator, you don't have a chance to see who will be riding on the elevator with you. (14) What you shouldn't do when you get your mail is stop to read it. First bring the mail into your home.   (15) If you think that your home has been burglarized, call the police from a neighbor's home. Don't enter your own residence, because the burglar may still be inside.

(16) Two good ways to make a burglar think that someone is home is to leave a light on and to leave the radio playing.   (17) To find out if a person at your door is really a salesman, ask him what company he represents and ask for his business phone number. Check this number in the phone book. If it is legitimate, call the company and see if the

salesperson is an actual employee. (18) To prove that the man at your door is really a policeman, ask him to slip his identification card underneath the door. (19) To avoid being mugged in an empty subway car, change cars and look for a transit policeman or a motorman. (20) For identification purposes, notice the mugger's shoes and pants. These are the two items that he is least likely to change.

(21) To get help when you have no phone, open your window and yell as loud as you can. (22) After you call the police, try to let the victim know that you have called. This way he knows that somebody hears him and that help is due to arrive. (23) If you see a getaway vehicle, you should be able to give police the license number, the color of the car, and the direction in which it was traveling. (24) Speaking to the mugger in a quiet voice may keep him from panicking. It will also distract him, so he will not be thinking about using his weapon. (25) With a dime or a quarter, you can call for help if you get to a payphone.

TEST 2: FIGHTING OFF THE UNARMED MUGGER

1. According to my definition of self-protection what is the purpose of using force?

2. When you decide to use force what is the first question that you should ask yourself?

3. When you are running away from a criminal what two things should you look for?

4. Approaching from the rear, a criminal places his hand over your mouth. What is the best way to remove this hand?

5. To escape from the one-hand wrist grab, what must you notice about the mugger's grip?

6. It is sometimes a good idea to cause a distraction when you are getting out of the wrist grab. Suggest one way that the mugger can be distracted.

7. How does the book suggest that you get out of the two-hand wrist grab?

8. The mugger's yoke is a stranglehold applied from the rear. The mugger has one arm around the victim's throat and the other arm underneath the victim's armpit. Both of the mugger's arms are joined. If you are caught in the yoke, what must you do to avoid strangulation?

9. Assume that you are in the mugger's yoke, what do you have to do to be able to reach the mugger's groin?

10. In Chapter 4, I recommend that if the mugger has you in a headlock, you try to startle him with a sharp pinch. Where should this pinch be applied?

11. Assume that the mugger still has you in a headlock. The part of your body closer to the mugger I will call "inside" and the part further away I will call "outside." Your next move is toward the mugger's groin. Do you step forward with your inside leg or outside leg? Do you use your inside hand or your outside hand?

12. When you are aiming at the mugger's testicles do you try to hit them or squeeze them?

13. In Chapter 4, I mention three ways to get out of the bear hug applied from the front. Name at least two.

14. In the same section, I list two ways to get out of the bear hug applied from the rear. Can you remember both?

15. Why might a criminal apply one of the bear hugs?

16. An attacker is in front of you with both arms straight and his hands around your throat. What must you do to break his grip?

17. If the strangler's arms were bent, how would this technique vary?

18. Think back to my discussion of the stranglehold. In what way did I consider this hold different from the other holds that we studied?

19. Is it safe to assume that female criminals are usually nonviolent?

20. I mentioned two parts of the female body that were very sensitive. Can you name them?

21. Suppose that you are attacked by two muggers. One is holding you and the other is striking you with a blunt weapon. It is necessary to use force. Which mugger should you attack first?

22. When you use a cane or an umbrella as a weapon, you usually use it like a bayonet rather than like a baseball bat. Give two reasons why it is **not** a good idea to swing a cane or an umbrella.

23. When would you not use a cane (or an umbrella) like a bayonet?

24. In describing cane techniques, I said that it is sometimes advantageous to back up against a wall. Why would this be helpful?

25. A mugger may not have any visible weapons, but he may still have a few advantages over the victim. Explain at least one.

Answers to Test 2

See how your answers compare with the responses that follow. If you are not satisfied with what you remember, you may want to turn back to the first half of Chapter 4 and skim through it one more time. Because of the importance of this material, you should look for a mark that is close to 100%. But even if you get a perfect score, it doesn't guarantee that you can use these techniques successfully; they still require practice.

(1) In my judgment, the purpose of using force when you are mugged is to escape from your attacker without getting hurt. (2) When you decide to fight back against a mugger, you must ask yourself, "What do I have available?" (3) When you are free and trying to outrun the mugger, you should head toward an area where there are other people and where there is little chance of being trapped (avoid dead ends and alley ways). (4) The best way to get an attacker's hand off your mouth is to grab the little finger and pull it back as hard as you can. As you do this, pull the hand away from your face. (5) To escape from the wrist grab, you must notice where the mugger's thumb and fingers are joined and pull your arm from that point.

(6) To distract the mugger while you are pulling your arm out of his grip, raise your free hand to eye level and snap your fingers. (7) When the mugger is holding your wrist with both hands, use your free hand to grab your own fist and pull it out of the mugger's grip. (8) When you are caught in the yoke, the first thing to do is to turn your head to where the mugger's arm is bent. (9) When you are in the yoke, your body is in front of the mugger's body. To be able to reach his groin, you must shift your torso to one side. (10) The victim in a headlock should pinch the mugger from behind on the inside of the thighs.

(11) To reach the mugger's groin while he has you in a headlock, step forward with your outside foot and then reach with your outside hand. (12) Squeeze the mugger's testicles rather than hit them. If a man sees a blow coming toward his groin, he will automatically flinch and there is a likelihood that his testicles will not be hit directly. (13) The methods I suggested for getting out of the bear hug from the front are: a thumb jab to the testicles, a heel slam to the instep, and biting any part of the body. (14) To escape from the bear hug applied from the rear, you can pinch the attacker near the bend of the arm or pull back his small finger. (15) The bear hugs are usually used to move a victim. The purpose of doing this is to either abduct the victim or transport the victim to a secluded spot.

(16) For the straight-arm stranglehold, you should raise your open palms to the level of the strangler's elbows and then drive the strangler's

elbows in. This will cause his hands to spread apart and the grip will be released.   (17)   If the strangler's elbows were bent, you would have to hit them from underneath and drive them up.   (18)   The stranglehold differs from other holds that I have mentioned, because the person applying this hold often derives unexpected excitement from strangling his victims.   (19)   Many people who are familiar with crime believe that female muggers will hurt their victims more often than the male. (20)   The female mugger is likely to be hurt if she is struck in the stomach or the breasts.

(21)   Ordinarily, if you are being held by one mugger and struck by another, you should deal with the person holding you before you turn your attention to his accomplice. But if the accomplice is coming at you with a dangerous weapon, you may try to kick him or avoid the blow before you try to get free.   (22)   If you swing a cane (or umbrella) like a baseball bat, you are *not* likely to hit your assailant in a sensitive area. Also, when you swing the cane, the other person has a better chance of getting it away from you.   (23)   You would not use your weapon like a bayonet if your attacker were armed. You would strike down on the attacker's hand until he released the weapon.   (24)   If you are using your cane (or umbrella) to defend yourself against a few attackers, it is important not to let any of them get behind you. To avoid being attacked from the rear, it is sometimes good to back up against a wall. (25)   The person who demands your money and has no visible weapon still has the following advantages. He may have a concealed weapon; he may have one or more accomplices; he has attacked by surprise; he knows what he is going to do and you don't.

TEST 3:   FIGHTING OFF THE MUGGER WHO IS ARMED

1. When you fight back against a mugger who is armed, you must usually do more than get away. What else must you accomplish?

2. Why will many muggers retreat as soon as they are disarmed?

3. Assume that a mugger is standing behind you and has a knife at your throat. Is it advisable to yell for help? What tone of voice should you use in talking to this mugger?

4. Once again, imagine that a mugger is holding you from behind with one arm and is holding a knife at your throat with the other. If you *must* use force, what can you do?

5. A knife is thrust at your stomach; how should you move your body to avoid being stabbed?

6. As the knife wielder's arm comes within range, you make contact with it to drive it off course. Do you hit or grab this arm? Where is the ideal place to make contact?

7. While the action described in Questions 5 and 6 is occurring, what should you be watching?

8. Following the action in Questions 5 and 6, I suggested that you poke the attacker in the eyes. While you are doing this with one hand, what should the other hand be doing?

9. Assume that you have grabbed the mugger's knife arm in your left hand and you are about to perform the wrist throw. What is the first action with your right hand?

10. You are getting ready for the wrist throw and both of your hands are on the mugger's knife arm. Your left hand must be moved. What will be its new position?

11. In the course of the wrist throw in what directions will the attacker's wrist be turned?

12. During the execution of the wrist throw, what body movements are needed (apart from the movement of your hands and arms) ?

13. Suppose that when your assailant lands on the ground the knife is still in his hands. What might you do to get it away from him?

14. In Chapter 4, I cautioned you about two things when removing the knife from the mugger. Can you name both?

15. Assume that a gun is pointed at your stomach and it may be necessary to use force. What should you be looking at?

16. You are going to try to remove the gun by using the wrist throw. You hit the wrist of the mugger's gun hand with your left hand. What is the movement of your body?

17. You have succeeded in performing the wrist throw. The mugger is on the ground in great pain. When is it safe to let go of his gun hand?

18. The gun is at your back and you think that it may be necessary to use force. There are two important things that you must find out. Try to name both of them.

19. To be able to see the gun, how should you move?

20. To disarm the mugger, you turn quickly. What is the position and function of your forward arm while you are turning? (If you are turning to the right, your right arm will be considered the forward one.)

21. Assume that the action in Question 20 is leading up to the wrist throw. What will be the function of the trailing arm? (This is the left arm if you are turning to the right.)

22. During the action in Questions 20 and 21 you have been turning. When should you stop and reverse directions?

23. Assume that you are with a companion and a group of muggers aim their weapons at this person's throat and head. What is your responsibility?

24. You are being robbed by a man who has a gun pressed against your head. At what point would you refuse to do what this man asks?

25. To practice the techniques of dealing with an armed mugger, what equipment do you need?

Answers to Test 3

See how your answers compare with the responses that follow. If you are not satisfied with what you remember, you may want to turn back to the second half of Chapter 4 and skim through it one more time. This test covers the most critical material in the book. Consequently, the techniques discussed require the most study and the greatest amount of practice.

(1) When you are fighting a mugger with a weapon, it is usually necessary to disarm him as well as escape. (2) Many muggers derive their confidence from their weapon. If you succeed in taking that weapon away, the mugger may retreat. (3) If a mugger has a knife at your throat, you don't want to make loud noises and panic him. Speak very softly, so he has to strain to hear what you are saying. (4) When the mugger is holding you from behind and has a knife at your throat, keep one hand in the vicinity of his groin. In a great emergency, you can reach back and squeeze his testicles. (5) When a knife is coming at your stomach, you must pivot 90° to avoid being stabbed. For extra clearance, pull in your stomach and throw out your chest.

(6) *Hit* the attacker's knife arm near the wrist and *then* grab it. If you try to grab it first, you may miss and accomplish nothing. (7) While the blade is coming toward you and going past you, your eyes should be focused on the knife. (8) To disable the knife wielder, you poke him in the eyes. While you do this, your other hand should still be holding the mugger's knife arm. (9) The first movement of the right hand in performing the wrist throw is to hit the back of the assailant's hand. This should force the wrist back and may cause the assailant to drop the knife. (10) Once you are holding the attacker's arm with both hands, move your left hand next to your right so that your thumbs are together and pointing in the same direction.

(11) During the wrist throw, the attacker's wrist is forced back and then twisted sideways and down.   (12) You are twisting the attacker's wrist and getting ready to lower him to the ground. You should turn 90°, so you are facing in the same direction as your opponent. For extra leverage, you can take a step with the leg that is further away from him.   (13) If the mugger is still holding the knife when he lands on the ground, you might try to kick him in the head to force him to let go.   (14) When you try to take the mugger's knife, be careful not to grab it by the blade and do not spend too long trying to get it. Too much time will give the mugger a chance to recover and fight back.   (15) If you look at a gun that is pointed at you, the mugger becomes aware of you intentions. Look at your attacker, but make sure that you can see the weapon out of the bottom of your eyes.

(16) At the same time that you hit the mugger's gun hand with your left hand, twist you body 90° to the right. This way if the mugger fires, you will not be hit.   (7) You should not let go of the mugger's gun hand until you have the gun. Even if the mugger is in great pain, he may still be able to use his weapon.   (18) To disarm a mugger who has a gun at your back, you must find out which hand is holding the gun and whether the gun is in range.   (19) To see the weapon, turn your head slowly. Do not move your body and do not noticeably look down. The weapon should be at the bottom of your field of vision.   (20) When you turn to disarm the mugger, your lead arm should be extended and a few inches above your waist. The purpose of this is to hit the mugger's arm and force the gun away from your body.

(21) When you make contact with your lead arm, you continue to turn and grab the mugger's wrist with your trailing arm.   (22) Once you are holding the mugger's wrist, you stop turning, reverse directions, and establish a hold with your other hand.   (23) When one or more weapons are aimed at your companion, it is your responsibility to remain still. What you don't want to do is to panic the muggers and cause them to use their weapons.   (24) With a gun at your head, the best course of action is to cooperate in every way possible.   (25) To make your practice sessions more realistic, the person who is playing the part of the mugger should have a rubber knife and a water pistol.

TEST 4: AVOIDING RAPE

1. There are two basic motives for committing rape. One is sexual gratification; what is the other?

2. What precaution should a woman take to disguise the fact that she is living alone?

3. Can you suggest three basic ways to discourage a would-be rapist?

4. If you are going to use force against a rapist, when is the best time to start to fight back?

5. Assume that you are on your back and the rapist is strangling you. To get him off your body, what action should you take with your hands?

6. The hand action in Question 5 should be accompanied by what other movement to dislodge the rapist?

7. As the rapist is propelled over your head, what can you do to travel with him and land on top of him?

8. Imagine that you are flat on the ground and the rapist has one hand over your mouth and one hand on your throat. You are going to use your hands to get free. What is your first move?

9. After you have dislodged one hand, what should you do next?

10. Describe the final part of this escape.

Answers to Test 4

Compare your answers with the responses that follow. If you are not satisfied with what you remember, you may want to turn back to Chapter 5 and skim through it one more time. Portions of Chapter 5 talk about the adjustment of the victim and her family after the crime. This discussion is not referred to in the test, but it is important.

(1) In addition to sexual gratification, another motive for committing rape is the desire to physically dominate a member of the other sex. (2) Women who live alone should not have their first names listed in the phone book or in a directory of tenants. Only their first initials should be used. (3) A would-be rapist may be discouraged from committing his crime if you convince him that you have a contagious disease, if you persuade him to meet with you at a later time, or if you make yourself unappealing by regurgitating. (4) If you are going to resist a rapist, it is advisable to use force as soon as possible. The reasons for wanting a fast response are: the sooner you get free, the less chance there is of being injured; you have a better opportunity to get away while you are on your feet; and the longer you remain inactive, the more difficult it will be for you to react. (5) When you are on your back and

being strangled, move your hands behind the strangler's elbows and drive his elbows forward.

(6)   As you are hitting the strangler's elbows, use your knee to strike him in the buttocks and push him forward.   (7)   As the rapist sails over your head, hold onto his elbows and turn him to the left or right. This will ensure that you land on top of him.   (8)   When you are on your back and your head and throat are pinned by the rapist's hands, lift your right side and roll toward the rapist. As you do, hit the inside of his right arm with your right hand.   (9)   Once you are free of his right hand, reverse directions and use the same technique to dislodge his left hand.
(10)   Once both hands are off your body, turn until you are on your hands and knees. Then crawl out from underneath the rapist.

TEST 5:   SELF-PROTECTION FOR YOUNGSTERS

1. I believe that teenagers and preteens are criminally abused more than any other group in our population. Why is this difficult to verify statistically?

2. Give at least two reasons why a student may not report a crime that was committed by another member of the school.

3. When youngsters are victimized, why do they hesitate to tell their parents?

4. When youngsters leave school late (after completing extracurricular activities), what precautions may be taken?

5. What can a school do to reduce the incidence of crime in its bathrooms?

6. What precautions can the student take to avoid being mugged in the bathroom?

7. When youngsters are robbed by gangs of youths, the desire to get money may be one reason for committing the crime. But what do I suggest is an even stronger motive? (Do you remember my name for the type of mugger who commits this crime?)

8. Suppose a youngster is walking down the street and his path is blocked by a group of boys. What do I suggest is the best course of action?

9. Name a few things that parents can do to make their children less susceptible to violence and crime.

10. Give three reasons why hitch-hiking is not a good idea.

Answers to Test 5

See how your answers compare with the responses that follow. If you are not satisfied with what you remember, you may want to turn back to Chapter 6 and skim through it one more time.

(1) Crimes against teens and preteens are not frequently reported. As a result, it is hard to estimate how often this group is victimized.
(2) Victims will refrain from reporting another student because they fear retaliation and they feel that informing is not desirable behavior. Many young victims will not want their parents to hear about the crime.
(3) Youngsters may hesitate to confide in their parents because they are afraid that their fathers will try to get revenge, that their parents may come to school, or that their parents will criticize them for not fighting back. (4) When youngsters leave school long after the rest of the student body, it is a good idea for them to leave the building in a group. If parents consider this dangerous, they can arrange to transport the students in car pools. (5) When school washrooms turn into danger zones, the school should have them monitored by security personnel or off-duty faculty members.

(6) If the school does not provide adult supervision in the vicinity of the washroom, students can go to the washrooms in pairs. One student will stand near the door, while the other goes in. If the student inside needs help, his companion is free to run to the nearest classroom. Before entering the washroom, the student should look around to make sure that there are no signs of danger. (7) While groups of youths may rob to get extra money, they are often more interested in establishing an image of being tough. I called this type of mugger the "status seeker."
(8) Assume that a youngster's path is blocked by a group of hostile teenagers. I suggest that he continue walking in the same direction and that he say "Excuse me" when he gets near the hostile group.
(9) Parents can help children if they teach them about crime at an early age, if they find out what their children are concerned about, if they don't discourage their children from confiding in them, if they instill in their children a mature understanding of the importance of fighting and image, and if they keep careful track of their children's activities. (10) Hitch-hiking is not a good idea because it is against the law, the rider is not protected by insurance, and the person who hitch-hikes is vulnerable to several types of crime.

• • • The answers to the quizzes have been written out in detail. You may want to reread these answers for a quick review of the book.

9
Conversations with Ex-Criminals

Throughout the book, I have described mugging as I have seen it. Much of my experience has been through the eyes of others. I have never mugged anyone and have never been mugged. Instead, I have learned from my interviews with victims and from my dealings with muggers. Now, in this chapter, I have asked three ex-criminals to describe crime as they saw it—from the viewpoint of the "perpetrator." Their recollections are on the following pages.

The information in this chapter was obtained during lengthy question and answer sessions. A transcript was made of these sessions and the most pertinent parts were extracted for use in the book.

Much of what you will read is in dialogue form. Where ever possible, the language of the original conversation has been left intact.

PETER SHIVERS, THE PROFESSIONAL MUGGER

Peter Shivers' first attempt at mugging was a disaster. His victim turned out to be a policeman. And, as a result, Pete spent a year in jail.

When he returned to mugging, he was determined to make it pay. He started to plan his crimes in advance and to make sure that his victims were carrying money. At this stage of his career, Peter Shivers was a successful, professional mugger.

Mugging was not Pete's first experience in crime. His first arrest was for possession of a zip gun. That came in 1937, when he was just 9 years old. He was put on probation, but he soon joined a street gang and his offenses became more serious—assault, grand larceny, and possession of a real gun.

Although there were 15 children in Pete's family, during much of his childhood his parents were separated. After Pete's early difficulty with the law, his mother felt that he was too hard to handle. She sent him to live with his father, and the two of them worked together to sell "King Kong"—an illegal whiskey.

By the time Pete was out of his teens, he had already spent three years in jail. His occupation was hijacking and he was extremely successful. He once cleared $40,000 in a single heist.

But Pete was finally apprehended by the FBI. He spent five more years in prison, and when he came out he was too well-known by the authorities to go back to his old routine. Instead, he turned to mugging. In the following interview, he describes his technique—his way of choosing victims and his ways of getting them to cooperate. Pete was a professional mugger, but he is now a counselor helping youngsters to stay out of trouble. In this sense, his is a story with a happy ending.

LG: What happened to you after you came out of jail for hijacking?

PS: After I got out, I met a friend of mine and he told me "Hey man, let's go out there and make some money. Let's go sting people." And I said, "Like, hey, that's not my bag you know." I had never done any mugging before.

LG: How old were you at this time?

PS: I was in my early twenties. We were up on Convent Avenue near City College. So we stalked a fellow. We were doing what is called a "double bank." I would lay back on a car and while the victim was approaching me, my partner would run up from behind. I would hit the guy and then go through his pockets.

LG: In other words, one guy would grab him from behind and you would hit him right away.

PS: Right, for the shock! And then I would go through his pockets and get his wallet.

LG: Did you ask anything?

PS: No, that wasn't my style. On my first time out we grabbed a policeman.

LG: Your first mugging was a police officer?

PS: And that sort of scared me. I didn't know what to do; I pulled the guy's coat back and here's this .38 laying there and his shield. I didn't know what to do. So I just told my partner, "Man, you got the police" and I ran.

LG: And you left him with the guy?

PS: I left him holding the policeman. So he got arrested, of course, and eventually they came and they got me.

LG: Did you do any time on that one?

PS: I did a year on Riker's Island. When I came out, I met guys who were really into heavy mugging. And the guys were telling me, "You don't make money grabbing people off the streets. To make money, you go downtown where the money is at." That's when I learned about the financial district in terms of how to spot your mark. Sometimes I would take a girl with me. She would go into a bank. She would pretend to be filling out a withdrawal slip or whatever and she would spot the mark. And when she spotted the mark, she would follow him out of the bank and she would notify me. I would be standing about one door away. She would notify me by giving me a nod and then she would hit the particular pocket where the guy had the money. If he had it in his breast pocket, she'd hit her breast.

LG: So, in other words, you were in a sense a professional mugger now.

PS: That's when I became professional, right. And as a professional mugger, you don't really beat your victim. You can scare a person just by voice—with a voice threat.

LG: Were you carrying weapons at the time?

PS: Not at that time. I was basically playing on the man's fear.

LG: At this time, what was your type of victim? Was it a female, male, young person, old person—or didn't it matter?

PS: It didn't matter, really. All that mattered was that they had the money. It all depended on how desperate I was. Shortly after that is when I got into the drug culture.

LG: You developed the drug habit. How large did that habit become?

PS: I had a pretty large habit. I really can't estimate the amount, but I can guarantee it was over a hundred dollars a day. And during that particular time, I went to jail for the last time. I got a five-year sentence for the sale of drugs. And during those five years in the penitentiary, I really started to take a look at Pete. And when I came out on parole, I saw a lot of things. I saw kids who were my friends' daughters or sons who had really gotten into the drug thing. And this is when I really decided to do a turnaround.

LG: Getting back to mugging, Pete, you told me about the double bank. Was that your main way of mugging individuals?

PS: At that particular time, I was able to go out and mug by fear, I would walk up to my victim and slap him. And I would say something like "Mother _____, you scream and I bust your mother _____ head."

LG: Did you do most of your mugging outside or inside?

PS: I would prefer to be in the street because I could see anything that was coming. Inside a closed building, I wouldn't know what was coming at me.

LG: How would you operate?

PS: I would usually cruise a victim [move him around], threaten him, smack him or her—whatever the situation—and cruise him into a doorway. Then I would perpetrate the crime and leave.

LG: Have you at any time carried weapons?

PS: I have carried weapons on occasion. It all depends on the area I was in. I found at this time that the Wall Street area was very easy in terms of victims. When I went into the Times Square area I would take a weapon. Because there you have some of everything. And like the guy may be trying to take you off. [The person you mug may be out to mug you.]

LG: Let me ask you this, Pete: Did you have the feeling that Whites have money or Blacks have money? Or did you have the feeling that you were not going to mug a Black because you were black? Or didn't you care?

PS: That never really entered my mind. The only thing that I shied away from was people who were lame. Also blind people. These were no-no's in this society at that time. Now it seems to be prevalent because it's being done. But during those days if you got busted taking off a person who was infirmed and you were sent to jail, you didn't have to worry about the cops. You had to worry about the cons, because that was a no-no.

LG: I bet you learned quite a bit in prison about how to mug.

PS: Oh yeah.

LG: Is there a difference between how guys and girls are mugging people now as compared to when you were mugging in the 50's?

PS: There is definitely a difference. I find today that the mugger is younger and more aggressive. I find that these guys really hurt their victims.

LG: You think they are more vicious?

PS: Yes. The trend seems to be toward more violence.

LG: So, in other words, where you would mug somebody on fear alone, you would say that these individuals are quick to hurt their victims.

PS: Right! When I actually hit a victim, I would do it to put the fear into them. But then if I saw that a victim was going to give me a hard time and panic me, then I would strike. Other than that, there was no real reason to strike the victim.

LG: Pete, you spent over 20 years of your life in jail and I guess you have done just about everything a young guy could possibly do. How do you feel about your life now?

PS: Right now, Grif, I feel as though I have a damn good chance and I am looking forward to having a normal life. I am going to get married again. And I feel that just to be decent is a good feeling. It's a good feeling when you can walk down the street and hear people say "Hi, Pete," "How you doing, Pete?" And you don't have to hear them say "There goes that God damn Pete; I wish somebody would break his God damn neck!" It's a good feeling, man, when you can wake up in the morning and walk out your door and greet somebody you know. And you don't have to fear nothing. And this is what I'm looking forward to. I want to maintain that because it's a damn good feeling.

JESUS TORRES, A YOUNG OFFENDER

In Chapter 2, I described different types of muggers. Jesus Torres does not exactly fit any one of my categories. He has robbed with members of his gang and is a hero to younger people in his neighborhood. But it would be a mistake to say that he commits crimes just to impress his associates.

Jesus has had a history of violence in gang fights and in prison. Despite this, I would not call him a predatory mugger. He has never seriously hurt any of the people he has robbed. But if one of these people had resisted him, Jesus might have hurt his victim without feeling any remorse.

His crimes ranged from the haphazard selection of victims in an apartment building to the careful tracking of shoppers whom he believed were carrying large sums of money. Thus, it is hard to look at his career in crime and see any definite pattern.

In one respect, there is a strong parallel between Jesus Torres and Pete Shivers. They are both members of large families. In the Torres household there were 10 children.

While Pete Shivers lasted through high school, Jesus dropped out in the ninth grade. He had not yet learned how to read or write. He looked for a job, but he was poorly qualified. Unable to get work, Jesus turned to mugging as a source of income.

Once he was into crime, he used the money he made to buy clothes and to help his parents. He gave money to his mother, but never enough to make her suspicious. Still she found out that her son was involved in crime. By the time he was 20, he had been arrested 24 times and had spent 18 months in jail. In the next few pages, you will read excerpts from his story.

LG: How old were you the first time you mugged somebody?

JT: About 16. My friend and I waited until a man came.

LG: The first person you ever mugged was a *man*?

JT: Yes. He was about 35.

LG: Did you hit the guy?

JT: No. I just grabbed him and my friend and I had a knife. I put it on his neck and I held him tight like this.

LG: The old yoke method?

JT: Yes. I used that so the man couldn't turn around and get me.

LG: Did you wear a mask?

JT: I wore a handkerchief because he lived around my area.

LG: Were you and your friend scared?

JT: We were kind of scared, but we got over it. We did it right.

LG: How did you know how to mug somebody? Did anybody on the block teach you?

JT: No, I just went to the dude and when he turned his back I grabbed him and I put the knife on him. And then I told my partner to search him.

LG: Did anybody on the block talk about how they used to mug people?

JT: A lot of people used to talk about it. But we never used to tell them who we used to mug. After that first time, we kept on doing it.

LG: How many times a week?

JT: I used to do it about three times a week.

LG: Would you take the whole wallet or would you give people back their papers?

JT: I would just take it and give it to my partner. He wouldn't search it; he would put it in his pocket. Then we'd get out of there. When we got around the block we would search it. We would take our time.

LG: What did you do with the wallet after you took the money out of it?

JT: We threw it down the incinerator.

LG: You said that you used to mug people in elevators. Did you have any methods that you used to use when you were on an elevator?

JT: When I'm in the elevator and I see a person, I look at him and he looks kind of scared. I keep looking at him and then I tap my home man.

LG: Oh, you have signals?

JT: We move our head. When the man gets in the elevator, he pushes his floor and I push a lower floor. When we get to that floor, my partner gets out and then I get out. My partner holds the door and I rush back inside. We usually carry this piece of wood to hold the elevator door, so the elevator won't go up.

LG: Have you ever mugged anybody outside of an elevator?

JT: Yes. We would stay in a building and wait until somebody came in. Somebody is bound to come in the building, you know. We could stay there for about an hour. And somebody would come. My partner would make believe he was tying his sneakers and he would be down on the first floor. I would be on the second floor. When the man got in the middle—half way up the steps—that's when we started.

LG: Have you ever snatched pocketbooks?

JT: Yes. But I don't like to snatch, because sometimes people scream. Now, when I need money, I just wait for people. I follow them. I don't care where they live; I just follow them.

LG: How do you know that they have money? I mean how do you know that you are going to follow them?

JT: I used to stand next to the cashier and watch. Sometimes I would have money in my pocket and I would go in and ask for change of a dollar and look around. If I saw a lady who had money, I would say to myself "That person right there." All I would have to do is look at the person and I would remember who it was. Then I would go back across the street and wait for the person to come out. Once the person left the store, I would stay 15 steps behind them. If the person turned around, I would bend down and make believe I was tying my sneakers.

LG: You would wait till the person went into the building?

JT: I would wait until the person went in before I would go in. Once I was inside I wouldn't have to look at her because I had looked at her in the store. I wouldn't want her to be suspicious because then she would start panicking and wouldn't want to get in the elevator with me.

LG: Jesus, let's talk about your neighborhood. Do little kids on your block look up to you? Do they know that you go out mugging?

JT: Yes, some of them know. Like almost everybody that hangs out on the block used to be into something. When I first moved there, I used to hear about the two guys who did the mugging. That used to be me and my partner. I never used to tell them that was me; I used to play along with them.

LG: What about girls? Did you ever have girls take anyone off with you?

JT: The girls used to take off the girls. We had a couple of butches [lesbians], and they used to take off guys too.

LG: What about youngsters?

JT: We used to see the kids go in the store and rob and we used to see them get caught. We would wait for them outside and beat the crap out of them, and say "You don't do it like that, man."

LG: So you told them how?

JT: We would tell them, "This is the way to do it" and then we would go back in and show them.

LG: So you actually had a little crime school?

JT: Yeah. I would say, "This is the way you're supposed to do it." Then I would go in and take it. And I would say, "Did I get caught! Look at you, you got caught."

LG: What would you say is the best place to mug somebody?

JT: I liked to commit the crime indoors. Once I would spot my victim I would follow them to their building and wait for them inside. Another good place is near a check cashing place. The trouble with that is if they see you looking around, they get suspicious. I used to follow people and when I'd get my money, I would leave and go home. I always used to go home and change.

LG: Jesus, you know I'm going to be using this information in my book and I think that what you've told me will help a lot of people. I'm also going to tell people that you know you've paid your dues and now you're turning over a new leaf.

JT: Right!

FRANCIS DUGGAN, A BURGLAR

In his first 26 years, Frank Duggan has been arrested 32 times and has spent 4½ years in jail. He remembers those figures because his frequent appearances are a standing joke at his local precinct. Frank Duggan is not a violent criminal. While he has mugged a few times, it's not his specialty. He once tried purse snatching, but the victim reminded him of his mother (now deceased) and he never tried it again. Frank Duggan is a burglar. He commits almost all his crimes when no one else is around. But that doesn't mean he couldn't be dangerous. When he enters a home, he carries a weapon for protection. If he was ever surprised in a home that he was burglarizing, the person who found him might be seriously injured.

For this reason, avoiding burglary is more than a means of protecting property; it is a way of insuring your own safety. From reading this interview, you should learn a lot about the way burglars operate.

LG: Frank, you committed your first burglary at 12. You were on drugs between the ages of 14 and 18. About how many burglaries have you committed?

FD: It's got to be close to 100.

LG: *100 burglaries?* Of all types?

FD: Stores, trucks, cigarette trucks, train wagons, cargo wagons.

LG: O.K. Let's concentrate on homes and apartments. How did you pick the apartments?

FD: Well, an apartment is a little harder than a home.

LG: Is that true?

FD: Yeah. But suppose a couple is divorced and the mother has children—or, even if she lives with her husband, he has to leave for work at 7 o'clock. At 8:15, she would be leaving to go to the school to walk the kids. So right there you have your chance. Or between 2:30 and 3:00 in the afternoon, they had to go to pick up their kids and you knew their husband wasn't coming home from work until 5 o'clock.

LG: Well, then you were casing apartments?

FD: Most of the time people would come and tell me. They would set it up for me.

LG: How would you gain entrance?

FD: Gaining entrance was easy. I would pick the lock or I would use a crowbar if the door felt weak or a heavy duty screwdriver or a tire iron.

LG: How long would this take you?

FD: To gain entrance would take me two minutes, because I'm forcing a locked apartment. The screws are coming right out.

LG: Did anything ever keep you out?

FD: If there was enough money and I wanted to get in there, I would get into your fire escape window with a rope.

LG: What about the high rise buildings?

FD: That's easier. You just scale them. Or you jump from balcony to balcony.

LG: Do you give yourself a certain amount of time to get in and out of a building or apartment?

FD: I always gave myself 20 minutes. If I couldn't get your door open within 5 minutes by shimmying, I wouldn't bother.

LG: You give yourself 5 minutes, not 20 minutes?

FD: I give myself 5 minutes to open your door; 20 minutes overall.

LG: In other words, you spend 15 minutes inside the apartment. At one of my lectures, you said something very interesting about dogs. You said you would go into a house even if there was a dog.

FD: It all depends. A dog will bark, but he won't bite. If I see a dog barking and he is wagging his tail, it means that he is friendly.

LG: So you look for a wagging tail and you listen for a bark instead of a growl?

FD: If I hear a growl, I hesitate. I'll take my jacket off and put it behind me and let him get the scent. If he bites my jacket, I'm not going in. That's an attack dog.

LG: Suppose you were in an apartment and somebody came in the door; what would you do?

FD: I would swing at him and run.

LG: You would actually hit him?

FD: I'm going to tell you something. A person can get a good glance at your face, but once they get hit in the head with a crowbar, they forget everything.

LG: Have you ever hit anybody, Duggan?

FD: No, I never had to.

LG: If you go to burglarize a place, how many people do you take with you?

FD: It all depends. If it is a private house, I do it by myself.

LG: O.K. We are going to get to private houses. What about apartments?

FD: For apartments, I like to take somebody with me, so they can stand in the hallway to make noise if somebody is coming.

LG: When you get in an apartment, where do you look for their valuables? Based on your experience, what is the best spot to find watches, money, or small items?

FD: Underneath the mattress.

LG: People still leave their money under a mattress? Any other places?

FD: Under the rug and in the kitchen in their cups. Also, I'll check the kitchen cabinet, the refrigerator, and freezer.

LG: Have you ever gone into an apartment where they had safes?

FD: For safes, I take somebody in with me who has more of a technique. He knows how to use a doctor's scope.

LG: So you have a guy that knows all about safes?

FD: He counts the clicks. But the trouble with safes is they take a good 15 minutes to a half hour to open.

LG: Let's talk about the suburban areas. What is the easiest state that you've worked in?

FD: Jersey was the sweetest one I ever saw. I usually like to work in this town that was not far from the bridge. I would look for empty milk bottles and a lot of mail in the mail box. Sometimes if I thought a house looked fancy on the outside, I would knock on the door and ask for directions.

LG: You'd ask for directions. Sullivan used to knock on the door and if somebody answered he would have a raffle book. He would offer to sell them a chance.

FD: I would never do that. I would tell people "I come from Manhattan" or "I come from the Bronx and I'm out here to visit my aunt. She told me to get off at this stop and I'm lost. She lives on something, something street." If there was somebody home, they would say "Well, I never heard of that street." I'd say, "Well, all right, I'm sorry. Thank you, anyway," and I'd leave. Now if nobody answered, I would go right through the bathroom window.

LG: That was your biggest entrance in a home?

FD: Everybody, everybody leaves their bathroom window open. I don't know why. It was so sweet, you know. And if the window wasn't opened, they left the screen with screws on it where you just pushed the screen with your hand, unloosened the screws, and pushed the window open.

LG: So you find the homes easier to rip off. Is it because people are more lax?

FD: I wouldn't use the word "lax." They have too much confidence. They put 12 locks and a burglar alarm on their door; they tape up all their windows, but they forget their bathroom. I hope people will read it in your book and straighten themselves out. Maybe once they read the book, they will finally realize.

LG: Where do people living in homes leave their money?

FD: Well, where I worked they left it right on top of the bureau.

LG: They figured nobody was going to come in, so you didn't have to look too hard. Let me ask you this: What would you, Frank Duggan, do to prevent a burglary in your own home?

FD: I think it's a good idea to leave a note on your door saying, "I'll be back in 5 minutes" or "I'm at the neighbor's house." Another thing I'd do is leave the phone off the hook when I went out. A lot of people get your phone number out of the phone book, call you up, and if you answer they won't try to break in.

LG: What about lights?

FD: Lights don't mean anything. You can leave a light on, but a professional burglar knows the trick already. He would go and knock on the door and if you answered, he would ask you something. But if your lights aren't on, he might think you're asleep.

LG: Did you wear any special clothing when you were burglarizing?

FD: I would wear dark clothes, but then sometimes I would try hard to look like the average person.

LG: Duggan, I'm happy to have you on this staff and I'm pleased with this interview.

FD: Maybe you'd best keep it out.

LG: Hopefully, it will help somebody; that's the main thing.

FD: It might teach somebody how to go into crime.

LG: Well that's true, too. But the other thing is it may help people to be more careful.

JOEY RODRIGUEZ, A DELINQUENT

The last portion of the chapter has been written by Dr. Estelle Fryburg, a highly regarded psychologist. She has provided us with a portrait of a young man who has participated in several crimes. She has drawn this portrait specifically for this book.

In these final pages, and in the next chapter, you will notice that the focus of the book has changed. Up to now, I have concentrated on the techniques of the mugger and how the mugger can be foiled. In contrast, Dr. Fryburg writes about the psychological makeup of one mugger and how this person can be helped. At first glance, this might appear to be a digression. But it is not intended to be.

If we can help a young man like Joey Rodriguez, we cannot only improve his life, we can prevent several crimes from happening. Helping Joey is the responsibility of the police, the courts, special agencies, and behavioral experts like Dr. Fryburg. But at some time all of these specialists need your support and understanding. It is my opinion that we should all encourage programs that help to rehabilitate a delinquent or a criminal. Such actions are not a sign of weak-ness; they are an important part of self-protection.

(As you read about Joey, you may wonder why so much has been written about his case. Joey may be different from anyone you know, but he is not unlike many underprivileged delinquents. By reading his story, you may learn more about young muggers and how some of them can be diverted from a life of crime.)

Joey Rodriguez (a pseudonym) is a juvenile offender who, according to his Legal Aid attorney, is a candidate for incarceration at Attica, a maximum security facility. Joey is tall, slim, dark-haired, handsome and soft-spoken, and it is difficult to identify Joey as the stereotype of a juvenile delinquent. According to the definition of delinquency the general public uses, "delinquents are the youngsters who steal property, commit serious crimes of vandalism, are sexually promiscuous and behave in other ways which violate the law." These juveniles are viewed by the public as the young people who are involved in wicked and antisocial acts which are outside the main-stream. Although the crimes of which Joey stands accused qualify him to be typed as a juvenile delinquent, Joey is not outside of but blends into the group of young people in the lower-class minority group neighborhood where he lives. His legal problems may in large part be related to his desire for acceptance by his peers and his participation in their activities.

Joey "hangs out" with the boys. He was implicated in an elaborate purse snatching and robbery of an old woman while he hung on the fringe of the scene watching the crime. Assigned to a probation officer, he didn't keep the assigned probation appointment, so Joey now stands accused of violation of probation. Other charges against him are cashing a bogus check, possession of a small amount of marijuana and a complaint from a girl who lives next door to him that he took her in the hallway and tried to force himself on her.

The judge, presiding at Joey's arraignment, assigned him to the supervision of Police Officer Griffith at the local housing police precinct. As Police Officer Griffith worked with Joey, trying to place him in a job, he found that Joey at twenty years of age couldn't read, couldn't write and couldn't even sign his name. Joey reported that he hadn't been in school since he was ten years old. At the police station, Officer Griffith taught Joey to print his name, began to teach him to read, and sought educational assistance for him.

Joey is not unique. Indeed national and international statistics report dramatic increases in juvenile crime each year. It should be kept in mind, however, that delinquency is that behavior prohibited by the delinquency laws, and that the laws are so broad that large numbers of youths (many of whom are not reported) engage in acts which technically qualify as delinquency. . . .

[There are many theories pertaining to juvenile delinquency and] the case of Joey Rodriguez supports elements from each of the theories. Joey's inability to read and write, lack of time perception (he forgot to keep appointments with the probation officer, the psychologist and his teacher) and generally poor functioning in tasks related to everyday life, led to educational and psychological diagnostic evaluations. The following are the findings.

Observations of Social Development

Joey is the younger sibling of twenty-year-old fraternal male twins. Both young men are good-looking, well-dressed and well-developed physically. They appeared to be accepted by their peers as members of the group when they were observed with other youngsters from the area.

Both Joey and his brother cannot read. Of the two, Joey appears to be more educationally impaired than his brother Johnny. Joey can only print his name, but Johnny can write his name in script, although incorrectly. The first letters of Johnny's name were written in lower case rather than in capital letters.

Johnny reported that he can travel if someone takes him to the designated place the first time. Then he remembers how to go by looking for the numbers on the streets. According to Johnny, Joey cannot travel, and has to be escorted to places outside the immediate neighborhood.

The Rodriguez boys had both dropped out of school in the elementary grades when they were ten. Both young men said that they had not been learning anything and "felt dumb" in school. Yet both indicated that they were most anxious to learn to read.

Psychological Evaluation

Joey Rodriguez has severe deficits in his cognitive and emotional development. The psychological testing reveals mild retardation and suggestions of organic impairment in a sociopathic personality. He is a very passive young man, highly influenced by his environment, with a limited capacity for making judgments about the consequences of his actions. He does, however, demonstrate in both his testing behavior and test results an interest in and a capacity for cognitive and emotional growth if given structured, individualized attention.

Joey's present overall intellectual functioning is in the subnormal range on the Wechsler Adult Intelligence Scale with a full-scale IQ of 64. His performance score of 70 is in the lower end of the borderline range; his verbal score of 63 is in the mental defective range. His lowest verbal tests showed that he has virtually no current ability for abstract reasoning or concept formation, very poor judgment about how to get along with people or around in the world, and marked educational deficits. His higher verbal scores indicate that he has motivation to learn and a good capacity for concentration on simple, structured tasks. His performance subtests demonstrate a reasonably good capability for working with concrete tasks and holding perceptual images, but rather poor hand and eye coordination. His higher scores overall in the performance subtests reflect his action-oriented, non-reflective approach to life.

Joey's perceptions of the world tend to be primitive: either they are child-like, simple images, or they are somewhat vague, confused ones. Sexual and aggressive impulses are easily expressed, with little question about their appropriateness. Gauging the appropriateness of such expression is something that Joey has not yet learned to do. He shows marked feelings of deprivation, a great need for caring and attention, and a consequent passivity and reactivity to others. One gets the distinct impression that he will do what important people in his world suggest that he do, with little sense of whether it is right or wrong. His own, internal controls are clearly underdeveloped.

The interpersonal world of which Joey sees himself a part is full of violence, fear, deprivation, primitive sexuality, and confusion. It is a world in which people act without a great deal of reflection, and will act violently more often than not. One gets the distinct sense that Joey has learned to trust people, but has had few people on whom he could rely for good examples of how to deal with his impulses. He shows some gender confusion about how to distinguish what is right from what is wrong. Things happen quickly in his world and seem to be somewhat out of his control.

Educational Evaluation

Joey is severely educationally disadvantaged for at 20 years of age, he is functioning at approximately a 5-year-old level in reading, a 4½-year-old level in spelling and a 7-year-old level in arithmetic.

In reading lessons which utilized the newspaper, Joey was able to gain meaning from the pictures and listened carefully to the others in the group read the story. He was able to remember some of the events reported, but was exceptionally poor in making judgments or predicting events based on the material which had been read. His comprehension of material gives one the impression of a young child (5–7 years old) rather than the 20-year-old young man he is. He can read three words: "cat," "see," and "book." He did, however, attend to the lessons and did not become restless although the lessons lasted for more than two hours.

Writing and spelling are onerous tasks for him. He appears to have poor visual memory of whole words and must look at the board for every letter when he is copying. It therefore takes him an exceptionally long time to copy words. He can only print his name, intersperses capital and lower case letters and sometimes misspells his name. He reverses numbers in writing, and cannot associate the spoken number with the visual symbol.

In arithmetic, he uses dots and his fingers to arrive at answers. The concept of "more than" is one which Joey does not understand. Joey appears to have developed compensatory strategies in his attempts to deal with the ordinary tasks of daily living. The instructor asked Joey to calculate the cost of three copies of the newspaper, and check to see if the correct change (55¢) had been received. He was unable to do the problem. He could not calculate the cost of the newspapers so he glanced at the price indicated on the paper (15¢), but could not arrive at the cost for the three papers. He was unable to equate the coins received in change (2 quarters and 1 nickel) to 55¢.

It is obvious that Joey is seriously deficient academically. At this point it is difficult to separate behaviors symptomatic of possible learning disability from the behaviors due to educational disadvantage because Joey hasn't been in school for ten years.

The educational disability would make it difficult for him to function both in the tasks demanded of an adult in affairs of everyday living and in employment. Shopping in stores, counting money, filling out forms for rent, utilities, and mail among other tasks would be a problem for Joey. In seeking employment, Joey would have difficulty filling out an application, traveling to the place he works, remembering the hour to arrive and to leave and reading simple directions.

Joey needs a highly structured, sheltered environment. Despite the handicaps he demonstrates, he has strengths which should be employed to help him master basic literacy.

The Prognosis

Joey is an excellent example of a lower-class young man who became involved in activities which mark him as a juvenile delinquent. An early history of learning problems in school, immature personality development, and lower-class social status appear to be typical of a juvenile delinquent.

Incarceration in correctional facilities does not appear to be the answer to the problems of these young people. According to Frank Tannenbaum, instead of diverting the person from a deviant career, such experiences tend to single out the individual as "bad" and may push him further into deviance. It is suggested that psychological and educational support services along with guidance from professionals such as Police Officer Griffith may be a far more productive approach to assisting young men such as Joey toward a fulfilling and law-abiding future.

Estelle L. Fryburg, *Ph.D.*
Manhattan College

To rephrase Dr. Fryburg's prognosis, putting Joey in jail will not teach him to stop committing crimes. In many cases, a young person in jail will learn new ways of breaking the law. When this happens, you and I do not really benefit from their imprisonment. We are not made any safer.

This reminds me of a conversation I had with Frank Duggan—a burglar who has been imprisoned 32 times.

LG: When you were in jail did you learn anything?
FD: Yeah, I learned more crime.
LG: What do you mean more crime?

FD: Well, this is the way it is; this is a fact. You see, Griff, you were never in jail. You don't know what it is to be in jail. But when you sit down with two convicts all you talk about is your past history in crime. And they tell you one thing, and you say, "Oh yeah, and you know I did it the other way." So, in other words, they are teaching you a new technique and you are telling them a new technique.

LG: Was that the main conversation in jail then? Did you talk about different ways of committing crimes or did you talk about going straight?

FD: Well, this is what the conversation is. When you roll in you always meet a homie from the street.

LG: Somebody you know?

FD: And you say "Yo, what are you here for? I am here for burglary; you know I burglarized a store." And the other guy may say "I am in here for armed robbery; I used to rip off token booths." "How did you get away?" I would ask. He would say it was easy. Then I'd tell him everything I do is easy. So he'd tell me his techniques and I'd tell him mine. So if I ever wanted to switch around and do something different I had a new technique.

LG: I know what you mean. Go ahead.

FD: Jail is mainly playing cards or watching TV. If you ain't doing that, you're talking about crimes.

LG: It's a school for crime?

FD: A school for crime! I've been arrested 32 times and I have spent 4½ years behind bars. All you do is go in there and you learn a new trick.

From reading Duggan's description, do you think a boy like Joey Rodriguez would go straight after getting out of jail? Or would he be likely to become more delinquent? I believe that this is an important question—not only from the moral viewpoint (caring about another person), but from the viewpoint of our own safety. We know that for many criminals, jail is not an effective deterrent. If this is true, is there anything that you and I, as members of society, can do to reduce the frequency of crime? The answers to that question are explored in the final chapter.

10

A Final Thought

In the "Foreword," Richard Ward said that it was unfortunate that a book like this needs to be written. All of us share his sentiment. But we also realize that we will never be completely without crime. The lessons in this book will never be obsolete.

While we cannot eliminate crime, we can take steps to lessen its occurrence. How can this be done? Avoidance, as outlined in Chapter 3, is only part of the answer. The rest of the solution lies in the work that needs to be done with the potential victimizer—most especially, the young delinquent who is not yet totally committed to a life of crime. Not all youngsters can be diverted from committing criminal acts. But for every youngster that *can* be reached, a potential victim will be spared.

I recognized the need to work with young people from my experience as a police officer and as a concerned parent. But I did not appreciate the importance of this mission until I was approached by a senior citizen after one of my lectures. Her first words were complimentary, "Great course, Officer Griffith," she said. "I learned a great deal." But then her tone suddenly changed and she said to me, "Don't you think it would be much more meaningful if you instructed *kids* how not to beat us up, steal our property, and disrupt our lives?"

Her question caught me off guard and my response was as much an excuse as it was an answer. I explained to her that in my lectures I try to deal with life as it is and not life as it ought to be. This ended the conversation, but the question that she raised still puzzles me. Can something be done to reduce the number of criminals who jeopardize the safety of our parents, our children, our neighbors, and ourselves?

There are many people who have offered answers to this question. Some popular sentiments can be summed up in the words "more police protection," "stiffer sentences," and "a harder line against crime." Perhaps this is the best direction. I am not qualified to say that it is not. But all of these solutions put the responsibility on somebody else—either the judges, the police force, or the members of the legislature. I still believe that in the area of crime prevention—as with crime avoidance—there are things that you and I can do to protect ourselves.

What I would suggest is that each of us try to reach just one kid on the street. What this would involve would depend on the needs of the youngster. For many underprivileged boys and girls from large families, just a little attention is all that is required.

In my own neighborhood as a child, this function was fulfilled by a man we called "Uncle Louie." Everybody, including myself, loved this man and looked up to him. He taught us baseball, basketball, stickball, and anything else we wanted to learn. The time he spent with me has never been forgotten and I have tried to be an "Uncle Louie" to every youngster I have met.

This does not mean that I have always succeeded. There are reasons why some youngsters are difficult to reach. I will discuss these reasons later in the chapter. But first let me present a part of a conversation that I had with a criminal court justice, Judge Antonio Figueroa. The judge is a man whom I admire greatly. I was reassured to hear that he believed that young criminals could be rehabilitated and that individuals (like you and me) could play an important role in bringing this about.

LG: Judge, is it true that you see more individuals between the ages of 15 and 20 than from any other age group?

JF: I would say that I see more adolescents.

LG: What about ethnic groups?

JF: I would say predominantly more blacks and then Hispanics.

LG: Judge, is there a solution to juvenile crime and, if so, what?

JF: I can only voice my feelings and philosophy on this. It has been stated by others who are more qualified than I. Until we hit the root of the problem—housing, jobs, education, and all the other means by which a youngster is going to want to achieve—we are not going to be able to do anything to help the problem. I take as an example a youngster who has 8 to 10 siblings in a rundown apartment, whose presence at home is not even noticed, who has to go out and discover life for himself in the street corners, whose going to school or not going to school is never checked by his parents or the board of education. He is going to look up to the hustler on the corner, who has a big car and a lot of money. This person appears to be affluent in the eyes of the immature youngster. While the youngster has this as his ideal, we are not going to be able to deal with him very well. But because a number of youngsters who come into this court are black or Puerto Rican, it doesn't mean that there aren't other youngsters—both black and Puerto Rican—who are achieving, and trying to do a good job. Unfortunately, we never hear or read about these youngsters, and we should.

LG: Many people say that "there are many people from poor families who don't get into trouble." Some say that *they* came from a disadvantaged home and environment, and *they* didn't get involved in crime. So, Judge, I ask you, is being from a poor family and a run-down neighborhood a valid reason for getting involved in crime?

JF: I believe firmly that a youngster who comes from a ghetto neighborhood, poor housing facility, and a large family with insufficient income, and on public assistance, is usually more likely to get into trouble than a youngster from a middle class, affluent, well-to-do, well-cared-for family.

LG: Judge, is there anything one can do to turn a youngster away from crime? In other words, Judge, what would you do to re-direct a youngster away from crime?

JF: There are a lot of things I feel could be done. I would first try to give a youngster a feeling of identity. A feeling that he is someone who can achieve.

LG: How would you do that, Judge?

JF: To do that, I would have to deal with the individual directly. I must be able to go one-on-one with him. That would be the only way I would be able to reach him, because generally he feels that he is just another individual. I have dealt with youngsters, and when I bring them into my chambers and I talk to them man to man, person to person, I get better results. The youngster knows that I take pride in him as an individual and that I am placing him in a position where he can be answerable to me. I say to him "now you are an individual and I come from the same ghetto: I had the same disadvantages and I overcame, but I can only help you if you want to help yourself to overcome."

When you put the onus or the burden on the youngster, although he might be immature, it gives him more of the identity and the leverage that he needs to feel. He can say to himself, "Hey, I'm someone; I can achieve. If you did it, I can do it." Of course, the reality is that he is going to find a lot of blacks out in the street struggling, but when he finds obstacles, he may think of them in terms of what he discussed with me. And I feel that is effective. I don't delude myself by saying that every kid that I touch changes right away. No! Some youngsters are harder to deal with because they don't have that kind of a mind and because they are too far into the wrong channels of society or our community. But I believe that we should try. And if you try, I don't think that you can be halted. We must all try.

LG: Judge, can a 16-year-old's or 20-year-old's attitude about crime be changed?

JF: Oh yes! I've been instrumental in doing that with the help of other agencies. Let's face it. I don't expect a 16-year-old to deal with the problems as I would, to see things as I do. And that is where the mistake lies. Some of our adults in charge of agencies, departments, etc. don't put themselves in the position of the individual adolescent. They should realize that they are working with a person who has not lived as long as they have.

So, as a general rule, we have to put ourselves in the youngster's position and then see how we can deal with his problem. In this manner, we can be more effective. However, let me put it this way, there are no easy solutions to the problem. But we must all try. Because the youngsters we work with are the future citizens of our country.

LG: Can we combat crime, Your Honor?

JF: Yes, we can combat crime if we all try together. We must do this without any hypocrisy, and that is one of our main faults—too much hypocrisy. People may say "If it doesn't touch me, I don't want to know anything about it." But nowadays everything has to touch everybody. Anything that happens in Kings county or Staten Island, touches us here in the South Bronx or in Manhattan. We are dealing with a community that is close. Transportation and communication have brought us that much closer together. If someone commits a crime in Staten Island today, they can come to live in the Bronx tomorrow and vice versa.

LG: You really believe it takes a collective effort?

JF: A collective effort of all the people. Men of goodwill must do it. We must perservere, because if we don't perservere we are in trouble. Remember we are dealing with human beings, not machines. The greatest thing the good Lord made was the human being.

LG: Your honor, thanks for this interview. I have always admired both you and your work.

JF: The feeling is mutual, Officer Griffith. I've seen the way you have been working with the youngsters in our community, and I am proud of you.

LG: I appreciate that, Judge Figueroa.

In working with youngsters, I have found that in most cases their families are unable to keep them from being involved in crime or in acts of antisocial behavior. This was not due to a lack of love in the family. The majority of young men that I have worked with loved their parents. And this affection was returned by their fathers and mothers. What was missing in the home was parental control. This appeared to be true whether the household was headed by two parents or by one.

What has happened is that youngsters are going out on the streets at an earlier age and are staying out later than they did a generation ago. The influence of the street has made the youngsters more difficult for the parents to direct or control. When parents lose their effectiveness, they must look to the outside for help. But what agencies can offer the necessary assistance?

Few schools are equipped to deal with delinquent behavior. If delinquency is called to the attention of the police and they refer a youngster to the juvenile courts, detention is the usual solution. But, as we saw in the previous chapter, detention seldom helps a youngster to turn away from crime. Thus, it might seem that if parents cannot control the behavior of their child, there is little chance of their getting assistance from an outside source.

This is a pessimistic viewpoint that brings me back to my conversation with Judge Figueroa. The judge appeared to be optimistic in his belief that youngsters who are in trouble can be helped. He indicated that the source of help should not only be the professional agencies but the community itself. He also stressed that the most effective way to provide assistance is to work with a youngster one-on-one.

Some people might criticize this approach. They might say to themselves "I took care of my kids and they grew to be fine young men and women, so let all parents take care of their own." This argument sounds convincing. But if we persuade ourselves that it is correct, then we deny the problem youngsters the assistance that they need. Another reaction might be, "The judge's ideals are fine, but they are not very practical. As a community member, what can *I* do to help a youngster who is in trouble?"

The individual will have to answer this question for himself. What I can do is describe my own methods and indicate their measure of success. Perhaps this discussion will give you some ideas of how you can be helpful in your own neighborhood.

I have been working with some 30 youngsters from various gangs in the South Bronx, New York. In my first contact with each of these youngsters, we came to an unwritten agreement. I offered to do my best to get the youngster a summer job or to get him back into school. The youngster, in turn, had to promise that he would stay out of trouble for a period of six months. The terms of this pact gave the youngster some direction. It also gave him an opportunity to prove to himself that he could resist the temptations of crime. During this six-month period, I tried to keep in close contact with the youngster's parents.

My work with these youngsters was reinforced by the support of my fellow officers in the precinct. These men befriended the youngsters and tried to provide them with a big brother image—the idea was to have the boys look up to someone other than the hustlers and the gang members who had gotten them into trouble.

All 30 youngsters stayed out of trouble for the agreed upon six months. Per our unwritten contract, all 30 were provided with summer jobs. One of the boys (case study Joey Rodriguez) left his job after the first day. Two were fired and one was arrested for attempted grand larceny—two months after his arrest, this same youngster was charged with the murder of a three-year-old. The other boys finished work. At the end of the summer, ten of them went back to school and the others went looking for winter employment.

It is too soon to measure this program's success. But I am convinced that it was well worth the effort. If we accomplished nothing else, we convinced these boys that someone outside of their home respects them and cares about what happens to them.

• • • This book presented the principles of self-protection. The earlier chapters showed you how to avoid being the victim of a crime and how to avoid being hurt if you ever did become a victim. This final chapter suggested that self-protection also includes the prevention of criminal acts. One way this can be accomplished is by working with youngsters. I have found this to be a rewarding experience and perhaps a sound investment in the future.